For Liz
September 1984

Paraplegia

PROGRESS IN REHABILITATION

Paraplegia

Edited by

Rudy Capildeo
and
Audrey Maxwell

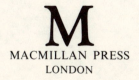

MACMILLAN PRESS
LONDON

First published 1984 by
THE MACMILLAN PRESS LTD.
London and Basingstoke
Companies and representatives throughout the world

Printed in Hong Kong

ISBN 0 333 34727 7 (hard cover)
      0 333 34728 5 (paper cover)

Contents

The Contributors

Gill ARNOTT,
   Senior Occupational Therapist, Robert Jones and Agnes Hunt Orthopaedic Hospital, Oswestry
Ida BROMLEY,
   District Physiotherapist, Hampstead Health District, London
Rudy CAPILDEO,
   Consultant Neurologist, Regional Centre for Neurology and Neurosurgery, Oldchurch Hospital, Romford, Essex
John CASTRO,
   Consultant Urologist and Transplant Surgeon, London
Gelia KIRKBY,
   Senior Social Worker, Spinal Unit, Stoke Mandeville Hospital, Bucks.
Ann MACFARLANE,
   Advisory Service, Kingston and Esher District
Tim MARSHALL,
   Lecturer in Social Medicine, Birmingham University
Audrey MAXWELL,
   Consultant to *Therapy*, Macmillan Journals
Graham POWELL,
   Senior Lecturer in Psychology, Department of Clinical Psychology, Institute of Psychiatry, London
Michael SMITH,
   Community Physician, Kingston-on-Thames
William Stewart TAOR,
   Consultant Orthopaedic Surgeon, Central Middlesex Hospital
Derek WILLCOCKS,
   Area Resettlement Officer, London North area

Introduction

Rudy Capildeo and Audrey Maxwell

'Ah, Mr. Beatty! I have sent for you today to say that I forgot to tell you before – that all power of motion and feeling below my chest are gone; and you very well know that I can live but a short time. . . . You know I am gone.'

'My Lord, unhappily for our country, nothing can be done for you', the surgeon, Dr Scott, said. Lord Nelson died within a few hours. A bullet had penetrated his chest and lodged in his thoracic spine causing acute paraplegia.

Recent events in the Falkland Islands have reminded us about our greatest naval hero and also the consequences of war and the inevitable casualties. It was in the context of war that Ludwig Guttmann was first given the task of establishing a National Spinal Injuries Centre at Stoke Mandeville Hospital, Aylesbury, which opened on 1 February, 1944. The unit had 26 beds and 1 patient. It was anticipated that the remainder would come from the spring offensive of World War II. During the course of that war more than 700 casualties with spinal cord lesions were placed in 12 spinal units throughout the country. Later, some of these units were closed and the patients transferred to Stoke Mandeville, the number of beds increasing to 100. By 1951 the unit had 160 beds and eventually 195 beds.

The contribution to our understanding of spinal cord injuries made by Sir Ludwig Guttmann and his colleagues at the Stoke Mandeville Hospital are to be found in his book, of which the second edition was published in 1976. So what of the future?

We must review our approach today, nearly 40 years after the opening of Stoke Mandeville Spinal Injuries Unit. At a time of recession and financial restraint it is very unlikely that priority will be given to the formation of new spinal units of the size recommended by Guttmann (1976: p. 46), namely of 50 beds, increasing eventually to 100 beds. One reason is that spinal cord injury outside wartime is not a common cause for hospital admission. In the United Kingdom the number is approximately 300 per year. Another reason is that patients should be treated, as far as possible, in their own community, because they must eventually return to that community to lead independent lives and to become accepted members of the community.

A few regional specialist units have been created with their own rehabilitation teams, but at district hospital level acute treatment and rehabilitation will be in the hands of a number of individuals rather than a rehabilitation team. This means that the 'average' doctor, nurse, physiotherapist, occupational therapist or social worker who has not worked in a spinal injury centre will have limited experience.

Progress in the future depends upon establishing new areas of expertise, training and research. In this book we have taken one type of spinal cord injury, paraplegia, and examined this subject from the point of view of the rehabilitation team. In this way we can see what has been achieved and what we can work to achieve in our patients. It is hoped that this small book will encourage a 'rehabilitation team approach' to the treatment of the paraplegic patient.

REFERENCE

Guttmann, Sir Ludwig (1976). *Spinal Cord Injuries*, 2nd edn, Blackwell, London.

1. Medical aspects of paraplegia

Rudy Capildeo

When the spinal cord is damaged, there is loss of motor and sensory function below the level of the spinal cord lesion. The extent of the motor and sensory loss depends upon this level as well as the degree of damage to the spinal cord. At the level of the cervical region quadriplegia may result; and at the thoracic region, spastic paraplegia. At the level of the lumbar spine flaccid paralysis occurs due to injury of the cauda equina. Loss of bowel and bladder function is common when there is severe loss of motor function. It must also be remembered that not all injuries to the spinal cord lead to paraplegia and not all paraplegias are due to trauma. For example, compression of the spinal cord from one side by a tumour may cause monoplegia or hemiplegia (see page 6).

Paraplegia should not be confused with quadriplegia — the level of the spinal cord injury, the resulting neurological deficit, the possible occurrence of other associated injuries, the risk of early mortality, the subsequent rehabilitation programme and long-term prognosis are all quite different.

TERMINOLOGY

There is some confusion in the medical literature concerning the term 'paraplegia'. It should not be used for any or all types of motor weakness in the legs regardless of the level at which the spinal cord is damaged.

Paraplegia is defined as complete paralysis of both limbs and *paraparesis* as incomplete paralysis of both lower limbs (compare with *hemiplegia* and *hemiparesis*).

Instead of 'paraplegia' and 'paraparesis' some authors use

Rudy Capildeo

the terms 'complete paraplegia' and 'incomplete paraplegia'. The term 'quadriplegia' or 'tetraplegia' is used to describe paralysis of all four limbs, and 'quadriparesis' as incomplete paralysis of all four limbs.

THE SIZE OF THE PROBLEM

Determining the number of people with paraplegia at any one time is very difficult for the following reasons:

(1) Do doctors in different centres, countries, etc., use the same diagnostic criteria for defining a case?

(2) Do patients in different countries have an equal chance of being referred to hospital, to a specialist, and of being recorded in a diagnostic index?

(3) Is the population under study (i.e. the denominator) adequately defined?

The first two points remain major obstacles in all epidemiological studies, making comparisons difficult. This is also to be found in studies on spinal cord injuries (Kraus *et al.*, 1975). If only 'persons admitted to a hospital with paralysis or spinal cord injury' are counted, then the overall figure, which would include early fatalities, will be underestimated. The approximate annual incidence rate of spinal cord injury on the basis of the number of persons admitted to hospital is 30 cases per million persons at risk per year. Reported incidence rates below 20 cases per million persons at risk are almost certainly underestimated. If all cases, including those based on autopsy reports, are ascertained, then the actual annual incidence rate may be as high as 53 per million population with a case fatality rate of 48 per cent. These figures come from Kraus and his colleagues (1975), who carried out a unique study in northern California comprising 18 counties, 5.8 million persons (29 per cent of the State's population), who had access to 184 hospitals. The study period was between 1970 and 1971. They discuss the problems of case ascertainment.

(1) Survivors of spinal cord injury are transferred to many different hospitals for various aspects of care -- emergency or

primary treatment and rehabilitation. There is a need for record linkage to obtain all the necessary data.

(2) In the diagnostic index up to ten diagnoses may be listed and spinal cord injury may not be the first listed on either admission or discharge indexes.

(3) Autopsy protocols may miss out spinal cord examination.

(4) Initial diagnosis may be inaccurate -- that is, missing the possibility of spinal cord injury or falsely mentioning the possibility. The discharge summary was the most important 'source of anatomic location and functional impairment data'.

(5) Examining death certificates without matching autopsy records will greatly underestimate incidence of spinal cord injuries.

Kraus and co-workers did find that 90 per cent of all cases could be found by studying hospital admission and discharge indexes. On the basis of their data, the annual number of persons with spinal cord injury in the United States was 11 200. Of these, 4200 will die before they reach hospital for treatment. An additional 1150 will succumb during the period of hospitalisation. The number of deaths due to late effects of spinal cord injury was unknown.

This study is unique. It provides the most complete overall picture of the problem of spinal cord injury and also helps to highlight the biases and, hence, problems of interpretation of those studies solely on the basis of cases admitted to rehabilitation units.

A further study from the USA (based on an incidence rate of 30 cases per million persons at risk) estimated that 8.88 beds per million population or just under 2000 beds will be necessary in the USA to care adequately for newly acquired spinal cord injuries (Devivo *et al.*, 1980).

The prevalence rate of people with spinal cord injury has been estimated at between 486 and 969 per million persons, with a figure of 500 per million persons being most generally quoted. With improved care of patients with spinal cord injury, many more are surviving each year. These figures mean that there are at least 100 000 survivors from spinal cord injury in the USA at a given time, of whom, it is esti-

mated, 35 000 will have a complete paralysis of both lower
limbs and 5000 will have a complete paralysis of all four
limbs.

THE NATURE OF THE PROBLEM

The study from Kraus *et al.* (1975) indicates that, overall,
quadriparesis is the commonest form of impairment (9.5 per
million population), followed by 'paraplegia, other forms of
paralysis, paraparesis, quadriplegia and other deficits' (7.7,
6.5, 4,7, 3.2 and 1.6 per million, respectively). 'Other forms
of paralysis' included hemiplegia, monoplegia and 'central
cord syndrome'. 'Other deficits' included 'transient paresis
or organ dysfunction'.

Traumatic causes

Half of all spinal cord injuries are attributed to motor vehicle
collisions, multiple or single vehicle collisions, and in the
study from Kraus *et al.* (1975) 20 per cent were pedestrians
struck by motor vehicles and motor-cycle collisions were
involved in only 10 per cent of cases. It is salutary to note
that for every person killed in a motor car 18 are killed on a
motor-cycle, and similarly for every person seriously injured
in a motor car accident 20 are seriously injured on a motor-
cycle, the pillion rider being especially vulnerable.

The second most common cause is falls, which account for
approximately 25 per cent of all cases, followed by sports
injuries, the commonest being diving into swimming pools,
rivers, etc. In the USA injuries from firearms are the third
commonest cause.

Non-traumatic causes

Non-traumatic causes include tumours, multiple sclerosis and
myelitis. Other causes are disc protrusions, motor neuron
disease, syringomyelia, epidural abscess, congenital malforma-

tions and vascular lesions. In the pre-vaccination era polio-myelitis was an important cause. Rare causes include subacute myelo-optic neuropathy (SMON) related to enterovioform toxicity in Japan and decompression sickness of deep-sea divers (caisson disease). Cervical spondylosis is an important cause of quadriparesis. The incidence of these non-traumatic causes of paraplegia is basically unknown. Patients will be admitted and cared for in a wide variety of hospital wards. Some patients might be offered physiotherapy but very few will be offered rehabilitation facilities.

Age and sex

The peak rates of paraplegia, quadriparesis and other forms of paralysis in males and females occur between the ages of 15 and 24 years. In contrast, quadriplegia in males and quad-riparesis in males and females show a bimodal distribution, with peaks at 15–35 years and above 55 years of age (Kraus *et al.*, 1975). The relative incidence rates are, overall, five times higher for males than for females.

Level and extent of lesion

The cervical cord is most commonly involved after spinal cord injury. A recent series of 359 patients (Fine *et al.*, 1979) admitted to a specialist centre at the University of Alabama indicated that the commonest levels were C4 and C5 rather than C5 and C6. In series from specialist centres, lesions at higher levels (C1, C2 or C3) will not be represented, since these cases seldom survive to be admitted to rehabilitation units. The overall impression from these data is that cervical cord lesions are usually 'incomplete', whereas thoracic cord lesions are more usually 'complete'. In a series from Stoke Mandeville Hospital of 100 consecutive spinal injuries (Silver *et al.*, 1980), 51 per cent were at the cervical level, 38 per cent were at the thoracic level and 11 per cent were lumbar. In this series the ratio between 'complete' and 'incomplete' cervical lesions was 3:2.

In the thoracic region lesions are commonest at T12, followed by T4 (Fine *et al.*, 1979). It has been suggested that the predominance of complete thoracic lesions may indicate a need for improved methods of stabilisation at the site of trauma and possibly during early acute management. On the other hand, it may be related to the amount of force required to fracture the thoracic spine rather than the cervical spine.

MEDICAL MANAGEMENT

Non-traumatic causes

The acute onset of paraparesis or paraplegia in a previously fit person is a medical emergency. In some instances ascending weakness of both legs with loss of sensation can be very sudden — for example, due to cord compression from an extradural mass or due to acute inflammation of the spinal cord or myelitis. A sensory level on the trunk is a very important sign. Myelography is mandatory and must be arranged as quickly as possible. If the myelogram indicates a spinal block, then expert surgery will be required (see Chapter 2) as a matter of urgency.

Patients who develop paraparesis as the result of a benign spinal tumour (e.g. meningioma or neurofibroma) usually recover very well after surgery and rehabilitation. Hemisection of the cord, a rare syndrome described by Dr Brown-Séquard in 1850, can be caused by tumour, multiple sclerosis or trauma. In this a spastic weakness occurs *below* the level of the lesion, a lower motor neuron lesion *at* the level of the lesion, and loss of light touch, joint position sense and vibration sense on the same side due to involvement of the posterior column of the spinal cord. On the *opposite* side of the body, loss of pain and temperature occurs, since these modalities are carried in fibres which cross the spinal cord to ascend in the lateral spinothalamic tract.

When paraplegia is due to secondary deposits in the spine from primary tumours elsewhere, treatment is very difficult.

If deposits are generalised, the treatment is usually palliative. Radiotherapy, steroids and analgesia may all be tried, particularly if the patient is in a lot of pain and discomfort. If the diagnosis is at all in doubt, then a surgical opinion should be sought as to the possible value of surgical exploration, with the possibility of partial or complete resection, biopsy or decompression.

Traumatic causes

Surgical management, orthopaedic and urological, is discussed in Chapters 2 and 3.

Transfer of the patient from the scene of the accident to hospital requires expert care. Delay in transfer and transfer by non-skilled 'helpers' may actually cause further injury to the spinal cord.

Management begins with a full medical assessment, with a history from the patient (if possible) and a history from witnesses. If chest injuries or head injuries have also occurred, necessitating emergency resuscitation, then it is all too easy to forget to take a history from witnesses who might come to hospital or, at the very least, from the ambulance crew who brought the patient in, because of the drama of the emergency situation. One member of the team in the accident and emergency department should carry out this task. It is also necessary for medicolegal reasons. A knowledge of the type of injury will help the clinical assessment.

Clinical examination will determine the level of the spinal cord injury and the probable extent of spinal cord damage.

Head and chest injuries commonly complicate spinal cord injury. In the series of 100 consecutive patients reported by Silver and colleagues (1980), 50 cases had head injuries, of which 41 were minor and 9 were serious. Severe head injury can mask the diagnosis of spinal cord injury. Blood or cerebrospinal fluid may leak from the nose or ears after fracture of the skull. The combination of severe head injury and tetraplegia has a very poor prognosis. A total of 32 patients had fractured ribs associated with haemothorax or pneumothorax. Chest drainage was required in 7 patients (mostly thoracic lesions) and tracheostomy was performed in 12 patients (mostly cervical lesions).

The clinical diagnosis must be confirmed by careful radiological diagnosis. This is a subject in itself. Missed injuries of the spinal cord are due to errors in clinical and radiological assessment, with the consequent result of mismanagement and greater neurological deficit for the patient. The cases reported by Ohry *et al.* (1980) are disturbing. In a series of 353 cases admitted to the National Spinal Injuries Centre, Stoke Mandeville Hospital, 15 patients had damage to the spinal cord which was missed initially (Ravichandran and Silver, 1982). In 7 cases the diagnosis was made after neurological or neurosurgical opinion, and in 4 after neurological deterioration in the patient's condition. Hence the need for repeated assessments in the first few days and also the need for a variety of specialists in the assessment team!

After all the initial activity, which might include the immediate treatment of life-threatening conditions, there is inevitably a lull. Nursing care is of paramount importance. It is automatically assumed to be consistently outstanding and never falling below this level, particularly if secondary complications (notably pressure sores) are to be avoided. The work involved to achieve this is often forgotten and seldom praised. It is during this phase that the other members of the rehabilitation team should be called in to meet the patient and the relatives, and to assess the patient. Fractures must be stabilised and further radiographic procedures, such as myelography, considered (see Chapter 2). The place of surgery must be discussed. Prophylactic anticoagulation may be required to prevent deep-vein thrombosis and pulmonary embolism.

The patient's progress must be regularly monitored and discussed at the weekly meeting of the rehabilitation team. Future plans will depend on possible access or otherwise to a spinal injuries unit. Waiting lists to such units can be 8 months or more, which puts all the emphasis for immediate care on to the *local* hospital team. If a place cannot then be found in a spinal injuries unit long-term care will depend upon the *local* community team.

Complications

In some patients *spasticity*, rather than helping rehabilitation, may cause a lot of problems, including painful spasms — for example, a patient with paraparesis ('incomplete' lesion) initially flaccid becomes spastic. Baclofen (Lioresal) can be particularly useful in overcoming this problem, the dose being gradually built up to achieve a suitable therapeutic response. Occasionally baclofen and dantrolene sodium may be more beneficial together than either singly. Fortunately, the use of antispasticity agents has virtually made surgical techniques unnecessary for the treatment of spasticity.

A rare complication of spinal cord injuries is heterotopic ossification (see Chapter 2). In a retrospective survey of patients admitted to four different spinal injury units in the United Kingdom and Israel, Goldman (1980) discovered 25 cases out of 738 over a specific 3 year period. The major factors were incidence greater in men; usually developing in the 20–40-year-old group; late admission to a spinal injuries unit (6 weeks or more); road traffic accidents; half the patients were complete lower thoracic cord lesions; high incidence of associated bony injuries, particularly fractured ribs; usually developed at one site; radiographic confirmation required, with 60 per cent confirmed within 12 weeks of injury, usually between 6 and 12 weeks. Patients with pressure sores were excluded from this study, since there is a known association between the two conditions.

Biochemical studies in these patients are essentially normal. Diphosphonate drugs (e.g. disodium etidronate) offer a real hope for the future and could be given prophylactically during the first 6 weeks after spinal cord injury.

The development of pressure sores is always a major setback and is a great potential danger to the patient. Treatment is a combination of patient awareness of the problem, skilled nursing, and medical and surgical treatment — that is, team work, with the patient playing the prominent role.

PROGNOSIS

Prognosis depends upon the underlying aetiology, whether the condition is acute or chronic, progressive or static, and the type of treatment possible. In general, paraparesis ('incomplete' paraplegia) or cauda equina lesions have the best prognosis.

Early survivors of traumatic spinal cord injury show neurological improvement in at least one in five cases in the acute short-term hospital and one in three cases after intensive rehabilitation in a special centre (Kurtzke, 1975). One in six cases with complete sensory loss and paraplegia show some improvement after rehabilitation.

The immediate outcome for paraplegics and quadriplegics is quite different in terms of mortality. As many as two in three quadriplegics may die within the first week or so after the injury because of pulmonary disease or associated injuries. Associated injuries are common after traumatic spinal cord injury and are the cause of half the immediate deaths prior to hospital admission and also of a major proportion after admission (Kurtzke, 1975).

In 1971 the annual death rate for traumatic spinal cord injury in England and Wales was 4 per million, in Scotland 12 per million and in California 14 per million (with an additional 12 per million with fatal injuries including spinal cord damage). Male-to-female ratios were between 2:1 and 3:1. Motor vehicle accidents accounted for between one-half and two-thirds of deaths and falls for between one-eighth and one-quarter (Kurtzke, 1975).

Life expectancy tables have been calculated for spinal cord injury victims according to age at the time of injury and the type of neurological deficit (Devivo *et al.*, 1980). The average weighted life expectancy for both males and females is 30–32 years, but there are important differences.

(1) Paraparesis ('incomplete' paraplegia). For males and females at every age, the life expectancy is virtually the same as in the general population — for example, age at hospital discharge of 20, 30 and 40 years in male patients is 47.85, 38.95 and 29.98 years, respectively, compared with 49.67,

40.61 and 31.53 years in the general population. These differences also hold up to 70 years.

(2) Paraplegia ('complete' paraplegia). For males and females the life expectancy is considerably reduced — for example, age at hospital discharge of 20, 30 and 40 years in male patients is 33.73, 26.29 and 18.55 years, respectively (again compared with 49.67, 40.61 and 31.53 years). This difference increases with age at time of injury — by 60 and 70 years, the figures are 7.08 and 3.93 years, respectively, compared with 14.65 and 9.00 years in the general population — and is worse for males.

(3) Quadriparesis ('incomplete' quadriplegia). For males and females life expectancy lies almost exactly between that expected for paraparesis and that expected for paraplegia, again worse for males.

(4) Quadriplegia ('complete' quadriplegia). For both males and females the life expectancy is much worse than for paraparesis or paraplegia. Taking the same yearly intervals, life expectancy for injuries at ages 20, 30 and 40 years in male patients is 21.57, 16.45 and 10.49 years, respectively (less than half of the general population figures — see above), with considerable worsening in ages over 50 years. Again female life expectancy is slightly better.

It is important to note that after rehabilitation following acute paraplegia four out of five survivors in England were employed.

For non-traumatic cases the prognosis is directly related to the underlying cause.

To quote Silver *et al.* (1980), '. . . the reduction in mortality has been achieved only by close co-operation with chest physicians and surgeons, anaesthetists and radiologists, by superb nursing and constant physiotherapy. Obviously one needs all the facilities of an acute general hospital and an intensive care unit rather than the ordinary ward in which our patients have been treated.'

Since the 'early transfer to the Spinal Unit' is not possible, the acute general or district hospital must develop the expertise and facilities to provide 'the crucial continuity of care from the acute phase to rehabilitation in the community'.

The advantages are obvious, since 'the speedy treatment of associated injuries and the prevention of early complications with the total expertise of the spinal team mean that the patient leaves hospital sooner and his whole well-being and life expectancy are greater'.

Finally, basic epidemiological data are still lacking. The type of study performed by Kraus *et al.* (1975) should be adopted to provide prospective data which would give a complete picture of paraplegia from all causes. There are no satisfactory published data on non-traumatic causes (Kurtzke, 1975).

REFERENCES

Devivo, M. J., Fine, P. R., Maetz, H. M. and Stover, S. L. (1980). Prevalence of spinal cord injury: A reestimation employing life table techniques. *Arch. Neurol.*, 37, 707–708.

Fine, P. R., Kuhlemeier, K. V., Devivo, M. J. and Stover, S. L. (1979). Spinal cord injury: An epidemiologic perspective. *Paraplegia*, 17, 237–250.

Goldman, J. (1980). Heterotopic ossification in spinal cord injuries. *Physiotherapy*, 66, 219–220.

Kraus, F. F., Franti, C. E., Riggins, R. S., Richards, D. and Borhani, N. O. (1975). Incidence of traumatic spinal cord lesions. *J. chron. Dis.*, 28, 471–492.

Kurtzke, J. F. (1975). Epidemiology of spinal cord injury. *Expl Neurol.*, 48, No. 3, Part 2, 163–236.

Ohry, A., Brooks, M. E. and Rozin, R. (1980). Misdiagnosis of spinal cord injuries – the physiatrist's point of view. *Paraplegia*, 18, 15–20.

Ravichandran, G. and Silver, J. R. (1982). Missed injuries of the spinal cord. *Br. med. J.*, 284, 953–956.

Silver, J. R., Morris, W. R. and Otfinowski, J. S. (1980). Associated injuries in patients with spinal injury. *Injury*, 12, 219–224.

2. Surgical aspects 1: Orthopaedic

William Stewart Taor

Most people would agree that in an ideal world all patients with any neurological disturbance following a spinal injury should be admitted to a special spinal injury unit, preferably within 24 hours of the accident, or as soon as the patient's general condition permits, in order to avoid early infection of the paralysed bladder and the development of other complications, particularly pressure sores.

Unfortunately, we do not live in an ideal world, and many paraplegics are badly or inadequately treated, owing to a lack of awareness of the seriousness of the original injury and the dangerous, life-threatening complications. It is well known that in many parts of the world ambulance and transportation facilities are inadequate and some hospitals are not capable of caring for the neurological patient. It is unfortunate that many paraplegics are dying, languishing in bed or in plaster jackets, with pressure sores and severe urinary infection, because of inadequate medical and nursing care and inadequate facilities.

INITIAL MANAGEMENT

The treatment of the patient with a spinal injury begins at the scene of the accident, with skilled handling by experienced personnel and careful transportation to hospital.

Wherever possible, the paraplegic patient should be transferred to the nearest spinal injury unit, but this may not be feasible for a few days. It is usual practice for spinal injury cases to be transported by ambulance to the nearest accident and emergency department of a district general hospital. The

immediate treatment of the injured patient is determined
along the usual lines by establishing the priorities:

(1) Initial resuscitation.
(2) Maintenance of airway.
(3) Diagnosis and treatment of life-threatening situations.

It may be necessary for an emergency laparotomy to
remove a ruptured spleen or suture a tear in the liver; to repair
a damaged diaphragm; or to insert a chest drain.

Fractures of the long bones should be treated conservatively
along the usual lines by skeletal traction or immobilisation in
a plaster of Paris cast. However, in the paraplegic patient with
multiple injuries and fractures of the long bones, there may
be considerable problems with nursing relating to the frequent
turning required and the development of pressure sores. It is
often preferable to dispense with traction ropes and plaster
casts, and to perform open reduction and internal fixation
of fractures, thus facilitating much easier nursing care.

From the neurological point of view, a very careful assessment is required, initially and at frequent intervals, to assess
whether there is any deterioration in those patients with an
incomplete nerve lesion.

The indication for emergency surgery in the immediate
treatment of paraplegia is somewhat controversial. There are
many reports in the medical literature advocating various
procedures, which include:

(1) Decompression laminectomy.
(2) Open reduction and manipulation of fractures or
fracture-dislocation of the thoracic and lumbar spines.
(3) Stabilisations, using bone grafts, metal plates, wires,
screws, external fixation devices, etc.

Emergency decompression laminectomy is performed
quite commonly in the Americas and the Middle East, not
only with the object of decompressing the spinal cord and/or
the nerve roots, but also to determine the exact nature of the
lesion. However, there is no real evidence that this approach
has produced any neurological improvement in those patients
with complete lesions, and occasionally neurological deter-

ioration can follow laminectomy in those patients with incomplete lesions.

It must be accepted that there is a tremendous emotive response in these patients and their relatives, and pressures are put upon orthopaedic surgeons and others to do something, if only for psychological reasons, 'for the patient'. It is my view that this pressure must be resisted, and each patient must be assessed on clinical grounds and the treatment planned accordingly.

Many case series have been reported throughout the world which show that a decompression laminectomy is of no help in complete paraplegics, and in some cases extensive removal of bone may cause positive harm by converting a stable or potentially unstable vertebral column into an actual instability, which may well require subsequent bone grafting and fixation procedures.

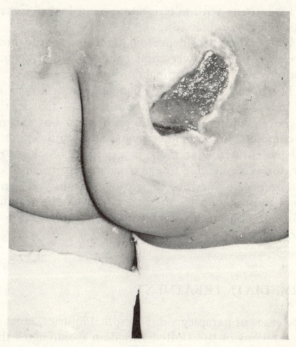

Figure 2.1 Pressure sore in patient with paraplegia and multiple injuries. Epithelialisation at edge of ulcer.

In the evaluation of the recent paraplegic, contrast myelography is occasionally helpful, although this procedure is not without risk. More recently, isotope myelography and computerised tomography of the lesion have been found to be a more reliable means of elucidating the degree and extent of the spinal fluid block, the amount of spinal cord swelling and the distortion of the spinal canal.

EARLY SURGERY

There is an occasional indication for early laminectomy in the following circumstances:

(1) In patients where there are ascending neurological signs above a complete lesion, due to an epidural collection of blood or haematoma.

(2) In patients with deteriorating neurological signs in an incomplete paraplegic lesion.

(3) Where there are depressed fractures of the posterior spinal elements of the vertebral column, with fragments of bone impinging upon the spinal cord or nerve roots.

(4) In those patients in which adequate X-rays of the region have demonstrated no abnormality — that is, there is no obvious fracture or fracture-dislocation but the patient has a complete or incomplete paraplegia, and where it has been demonstrated that there is a definite block on myelography, for example, due to a massive disc protrusion.

(5) The development of increasing neurological signs after a normal period, due to an aggravation by the trauma of a pre-existing condition — for example, spinal tumour or chronic infection.

INTERMEDIATE TREATMENT

In those cases of paraplegia due to spinal injuries, most orthopaedic surgeons in the United Kingdom would agree that for the vertebral injury the treatment of choice is by *prolonged immobilisation* and *postural reduction* of the fractures or fracture-dislocation on a special bed which permits regular turning and skin protection.

Because of lack of facilities and inadequate resources in some countries, many paraplegics are treated for many months and sometimes years in plaster of Paris beds and jackets. We recognise that this is a very dangerous situation, and that recumbency and prolonged immobilisation will inevitably lead to osteoporosis, pressure sores, bladder problems and contractures.

There is some controversy regarding the place of operative treatment to stabilise the spine in *early* cases of paraplegia with fractures or fracture-dislocation of the vertebral column. Many papers have been written in the past, and recent literature also advocates a variety of procedures to stabilise the spine, but there is no real evidence that there is any long-term advantage.

My approach to the treatment of fractures and fracture-dislocation is 8–12 weeks of postural reduction on a turning bed with X-ray examination at intervals. In common with Bedbrook (1971), Guttman (1976) and others, my experience is that the great majority of spinal injuries have gone on to a natural fusion by this time, when it would be safe to mobilise the patient in a wheelchair. If there is X-ray evidence of delayed union of the fractures or fracture-dislocation, a polythene or Plastazote jacket can be used for a short time in order to avoid excessive movements. X-rays taken at intervals would determine when the wearing of the jacket or corset should be discontinued.

There is an occasional indication for spinal fusion operations where stability has not been achieved by conservative measures, and where there is localised pain at the fracture site, increasing angular or rotational deformity, and where difficulty is experienced with the mobilisation of the patient in a wheelchair. A variety of techniques has been described which depend upon the experience of the orthopaedic surgeon and the facilities available -- for example, stabilisation of the spine by use of wires, rigid metal plates and rods; and bone grafts placed either anteriorly, anterolateral or via a posterior approach. There are disadvantages attached to the use of metal plates, and the Harrington system of distraction rods and hooks which produce a long rigid spinal segment. This can occasionally cause pain, and if there is loosening of the fixation device, a further operation will be necessary to remove the metal parts.

In the late case where stability has not been achieved, my approach is to use an anterolateral spinal fusion with extensive cortico-cancellous bone grafts and no rigid internal fixation with plates or rods. Following the bone graft operation, there is a further period of immobilisation on a turning bed for up to 3 months until a sound bony fusion has occurred. It is sometimes necessary to combine an anterior and a posterior bone graft operation to obtain the necessary sound bony fusion of an unstable fracture-dislocation.

LATE MANAGEMENT

The essence of treatment of the established paraplegic is prevention, the rehabilitation team working together to prevent complications such as pressure sores, spasticity and contractures. If the system of prevention breaks down, it may then be necessary for the orthopaedic surgeon to become involved in the management of these complications.

Osteoporosis

In paraplegics osteoporosis or loss of bone stock occurs in the lower limbs following a period of prolonged bed rest, especially when combined with immobilisation, and the condition is aggravated by chronic infection of the urinary tract and from pressure sores. Prevention of the condition is by early mobilisation and ambulation of the patient.

Osteoporotic bone is more brittle, and it is possible to get pathological or 'spontaneous' fractures following minor trauma or during passive movements of the leg by a physiotherapist. An impacted supracondylar fracture of the femur is a typical fracture sustained by paraplegics from falling out of a wheelchair on to the knee. These fractures are often

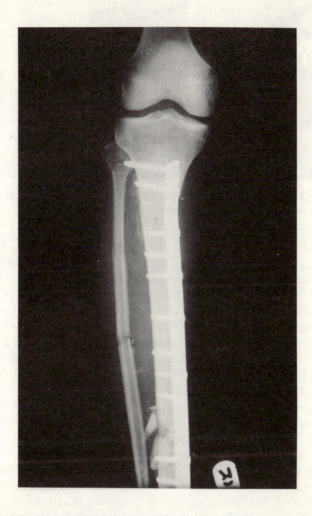

Figure 2.2 Anteroposterior X-ray of right lower leg showing internal fixation of comminuted tibial fracture.

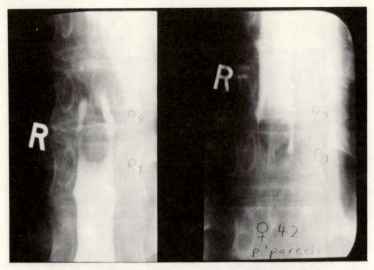

Figure 2.3 Myelogram demonstrating almost complete block at D8-9 due to massive dorsal disc protrusion.

missed, as the patient does not experience any pain. However, the appearance in a limb of localised swelling with increased heat, abnormal mobility and clicking should draw attention to a possible fracture.

The aim of treatment of osteoporosis is to mobilise as soon as possible by frequent and regular changes of position. The treatment of pathological osteoporotic fractures is, as a rule, conservative, by applying splints or plasters, although care should be taken to prevent the development of pressure sores. However, there are problems following the conservative management of these fractures, in that inevitably there is a further period of immobilisation with further osteoporosis; and in the presence of spasticity, complications may occur, with malunion of the fractures with associated angular or rotational deformities of the limbs. On occasions, correct immobilisation and alignment may not be possible, owing to marked spasticity. If at all possible, it is preferable to treat these pathological fractures by early open reduction and rigid internal fixation followed by early mobilisation and a return to the programme of rehabilitation.

Heterotopic ossification

An unusual form of extra-articular, extracapsular new bone ossification is seen occasionally following head and spinal injuries. The cause of this condition is obscure, but it does not appear to be related to overenthusiastic physiotherapy. The para-articular ossification occurs commonly around the

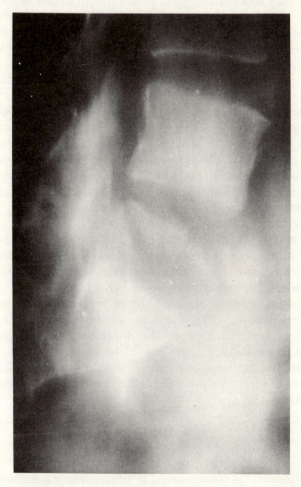

Figure 2.4 Lateral X-ray of lower lumbar spine, illustrating typical anterior tuberculosis involving body 5th lumbar vertebra.

hip, knee and elbow joints, but the articular surfaces remain unaffected. The ossification can become so massive, especially round the hip joints, that there is an effective extra-articular bony ankylosis which, if it develops with the hip in full extension, may well prevent the patient from sitting in a wheelchair.

The heterotopic new bone develops slowly, and it may take 18-24 months before it is mature. In a number of cases it has been possible to excise partially or completely this heterotopic ossification from around the hip joint, restoring hip flexion so that patients could then sit in a wheelchair. Unfortunately, if the new bone is excised too early, it often recurs. All workers interested in this unusual condition are agreed that excision of the heterotopic ossification should only be performed when the process of ossification has been completed. Recently various investigations have been carried out in an attempt to determine the maturity of the heterotopic ossification by assessing alkaline phosphatase values and using radioisotope scanning, but at the present time there is no reliable indicator for determining that the heterotopic ossification has reached maturity, thus indicating the most suitable time for surgical excision.

Stover *et al.* (1976) found that one of the diphosphonate drugs, disodium etidronate, was effective in the prevention of postoperative recurrence of heterotopic ossification in patients with spinal cord injuries. It has been shown that the diphosphonate drugs delayed the recurrence of the heterotopic ossification while the drugs were being taken, but the new bone came back when the drugs were stopped. At the present time further trials are being conducted, and it is possible that diphosphonate drugs should be taken following spinal cord injury to prevent the development of heterotopic ossification.

Care of the skin

Prevention of pressure sores is of paramount importance from day 1 following the accident. Sores can develop in any situation where there is pressure, but there are certain areas of the body which are more vulnerable, such as the sacrum, greater trochanters, ischium, knees, heels and toes. Deep pressure sores involving fascia, muscle and bone may communicate with bursae or joints. Pressure sores may be further complicated by infection, osteomyelitis and septicaemia.

Treatment of the established pressure sore has been well described by Guttmann (1976). The essence of treatment is

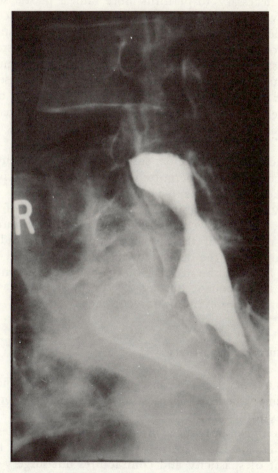

Figure 2.5 Lateral myelogram X-ray of same patient as in figure 2.4, showing anterior compression of the column due to caseous material and tuberculous pus.

excision of slough and necrotic tissue, free drainage of infected cavities, and appropriate dressings to promote granulations and epithelialisation. Healing can often be accelerated surgically by skin grafts once the granulations have reached the level of the surrounding skin. Large skin defects are covered with pinch grafts or split skin grafts. In areas where there are thin scars which frequently break down under pressure it may be necessary to perform more radical plastic surgery. A great variety of rotation and transposition flaps containing whole thickness of skin and subcutaneous tissue have been advocated for the surgical repair of large sores, especially over the sacrum and the greater trochanters of the femur.

In situations where there are very deep sinuses and neglected trochanteric or ischial sores resulting in chronic osteomyelitis of bone, more radical surgery may be required, with excision of the ischium or the head and neck of the femur.

Advances in microvascular surgery and the use of the operating microscope have permitted the use of better-vascularised and thicker muscle flaps to cover large skin defects.

Finally, it should be reiterated that the healing of a pressure sore, whether by conservative or surgical procedures, will not be successful if the patient has not received adequate instruction about the dangers of further pressure and how to avoid it. It cannot be stressed too strongly that prevention of pressure and frequent turning are the most important precondition in the prevention or recurrence of sores.

Contractures and spasticity

Contractures develop as a consequence of spasticity, incorrect positioning in bed or poor posture in a wheelchair, or inadequate physiotherapy.

Spasticity can be reduced in a number of ways (as described in Chapter 1). There are many surgical procedures for the treatment of spasticity and contractures but surgery on the spinal cord or nerve roots is no longer justified for traumatic lesions of the spinal cord. Tenotomies, myotomies, nerve resection, osteotomies and other surgical procedures on the peripheral structures have all been used. In my experience the following procedures may be useful in selected cases:

(1) Abdominal extraperitoneal obturator neurectomy where there is very troublesome adductor spasm and contractures associated with a scissor gait and difficulties with personal hygiene and nursing care. This operation is often combined with an adductor and iliopsoas release.

(2) Elongation of the tendo Achilles, usually by the White slide technique. Occasionally, this procedure is combined with a tibialis posterior tenotomy or transposition to the dorsal aspect of the foot.

(3) Resection of the inner hamstring tendons, with or without elongation of the biceps femoris tendon, to correct spasticity and flexor contracture at the knee to restore standing and walking.

NON-TRAUMATIC PARAPLEGIA

Although the number of paraplegics from road traffic and sporting accidents are increasing, it should be remembered that in the Third World the majority of patients presenting with paraplegia, especially those with incomplete lesions, are due to non-traumatic causes (see Chapter 1) — for example, tumours, disc prolapses, and epidural abscesses, commonly due to tuberculosis.

Whereas there has been a fall in the national incidence of tuberculosis in the UK, in the London Borough of Brent there has been a marked increase in tuberculosis over the course of the last 10 years, and approximately 12 per cent of these cases have involved the bones and joints. This increase in tuberculosis has coincided with the influx of Asian and Afro-Asian immigrants.

In the series of bone and joint tuberculosis in Brent, just over 50 per cent of cases had vertebral column involvement and approximately 30 per cent of these cases had neurological signs, with developing tetraplegia and paraplegia.

In recent years there has been an increase in the number of patients presenting with neurological signs in the lower limbs due to tuberculous osteomyelitis of the spine. A different treatment routine is required. The usual deformity in spinal tuberculosis is anterior, with vertebral body collapse, and tuberculous pus and caseous material tracks backwards, compressing the spinal canal from the front. Until 1976-7, my

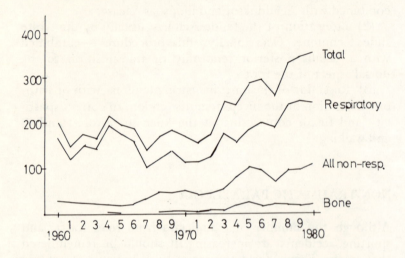

Figure 2.6 Graph to demonstrate increased tuberculosis notifications in Brent.

approach was to treat patients with anterior spinal disease and neurological signs along the established orthopaedic lines, by operative surgery — often radical surgery by an anterior or anterolateral decompression, débridement of all the tuberculous material and dead bone, followed by stabilisation using bone grafts.

Many authors have quite rightly condemned laminectomy in the treatment of spinal tuberculosis on the grounds that the disease is anterior and that, following the decompression and excision of the posterior bony elements, the vertebral column is rendered unstable, necessitating a prolonged period of immobilisation or further surgical treatment to stabilise the spine. In all previous series on spinal tuberculosis it has

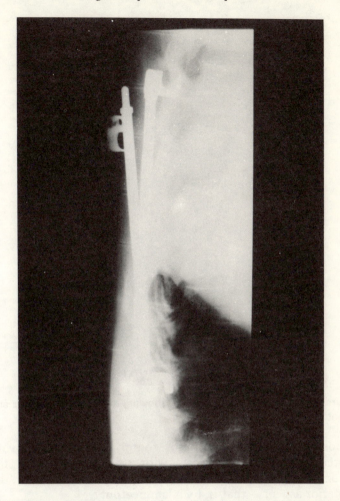

Figure 2.7 Lateral X-ray spinal fusion with Harrington rods with one lower clip cut out and loose rod.

been noted that there were 5 per cent of atypical spinal lesions. However, in the more recent Brent series of cases there have been approximately 25 per cent atypical lesions, with involvement of the posterior and posterolateral elements of the vertebral column, and, most importantly, there is compression of the spinal cord or nerve roots from the back, as

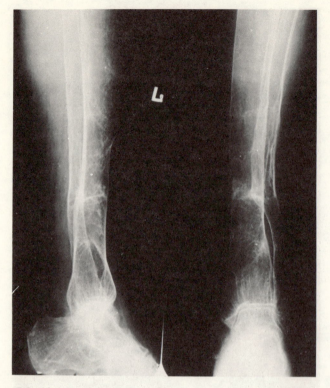

Figure 2.8 X-rays of the lower leg, showing marked osteoporosis and 'spontaneous fractures'.

opposed to the usual anterior route. In those cases with posterior spinal tuberculosis with neurological signs, the decompression operation should be performed from the posterior aspect — that is, by a laminectomy.

With the advance in chemotherapy, improved diagnostic aids, early diagnosis and confidence, from 1977 we have changed our treatment policy. Surgical treatment of spinal tuberculosis is rarely necessary except in the following indications:

(1) Progressive deterioration in the neurological picture.
(2) Very large abscesses.
(3) To obtain material for bacteriological and histological examination to confirm the diagnosis.

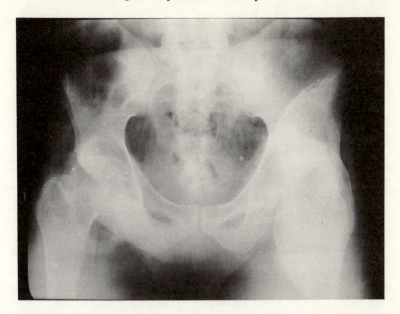

Figure 2.9 Anteroposterior X-ray of pelvis, showing extensive hetero-topic ossification of the hips and large bladder calculi.

After a period of initial assessment in hospital, all patients with spinal tuberculosis are treated on an ambulant, out-patient basis, with no period of immobilisation in plaster beds and without any form of external support from plaster jackets or lumbar corsets. All patients are treated with the modern antituberculous drugs, with a combination of three drugs (isoniazid, rifampicin and pyrazinamide) for 3 months and then isoniazid and rifampicin for a further 9–15 months.

In those cases of spinal tuberculosis where there is neuro-logical deterioration, I have advised an anterior or antero-lateral decompression operation if the vertebral bodies are involved, and a decompression laminectomy if the tuberculous disease involves the posterior or posterolateral elements.

In the management of the paraplegic patient it is important to know what the orthopaedic surgeon has to offer and when he could help. An early opinion soon after the onset of para-plegia as to the value or otherwise of surgery will help to allay the anxieties of the patient and relatives that everything possible has been considered.

REFERENCES

Bedbrook, G. (1971). Stability of spinal fractures and fracture dislocations. *Paraplegia*, 9, 23-32.
Guttmann, Sir L. (1976). *Spinal Cord Injuries*, 2nd edn, Blackwell, London.
Stover, S. L., Niemann, K. M. W. and Miller, J. M. (1976). Disodium etidronate in the prevention of postoperative recurrence of heterotopic ossification in spinal cord injury patients. *J. Bone Jt Surg.*, 58A, 683.

3. Surgical aspects 2: Urological

John Castro

The long-term survival of patients with spinal cord damage depends upon many factors, but most important is the management of the urinary tract and the avoidance of complications which ultimately lead to progressive renal damage. Renal failure is the most common cause of death among spinal injury patients who survive the early complications.

NORMAL BLADDER FUNCTION

To understand the effects of paraplegia on the bladder, it is necessary to consider the factors normally concerned in micturition. The empty bladder fills at an average rate of approximately 1 ml/min by a series of small squirts of urine from the ureters. The urine within the resting bladder is held at the bladder neck and there is little tension within the bladder wall, which, at this stage, conforms its shape to the surrounding structures. Pressure in the filling bladder remains at approximately 10 cm of water when prone but rises to 20 cm water when the subject is sitting or standing, probably because of the weight of abdominal organs. During a cough or when the subject strains, the pressure rises to 150 cm water. However, in normals there is no urinary leakage. This is because during coughing the perineal muscles also contract and so increase the resistance to voiding. There is also no detrusor (bladder wall) contraction and, hence, micturition is not initiated.

As the bladder continues to fill to capacity, it sends messages to the micturition centre in the brain and the brain responds with inhibitory signals to the bladder. Normally the patient is unaware of the bladder filling.

When urination is desired and it is socially acceptable, the bladder wall tension increases and abdominal straining occurs, thereby increasing intravesical pressure. When pressure reaches 60-70 cm water, urine flow begins and the urethra opens maximally. Urine flow rate and intravesical pressure increase smoothly. Any rapid changes are due to voluntary contractions of abdominal or perineal muscles. Towards the end of voiding bladder pressure and flow both fall.

NEUROLOGICAL PATHWAYS CONCERNED WITH MICTURITION

Micturition is basically a function of the autonomic nervous system which subsequently comes under the voluntary control of the cerebral hemispheres.

The sacral autonomic centre for micturition is in the caudal part of the spinal cord, called the conus medullaris. The neurons concerned are in the 3rd sacral segment and commonly extend into the 2nd segment. Occasionally they spread to the 4th and 5th segments. All of the reflexes between mucosa of the bladder and urethra, and the non-striated and striated muscles of the pelvic floor and urogenital diaphragm are organised in these segments. All of the nerve fibres to and from the brain concerned with bladder function come from and go to the conus. The parasympathetic fibres that supply the detrusor, perineal muscles and external sphincters also arise in these segments. In addition to the parasympathetic system and somatic musculature already described, the sympathetic nervous system plays a role in the function of the bladder. This system is located between the 1st thoracic and 3rd lumbar segments inclusive.

In order to exercise voluntary control on the bladder, it is necessary for the central nervous system to be continuously supplied with information concerning the progress of the actions it is carrying out. Afferent pathways from the bladder run in the pelvic nerves to the spinal cord; in the spinal cord the spinothalamic tract is the pathway conveying information to the cerebral cortex and it makes us aware of vesical events and gives the sensation underlying the desire to micturate.

Within the spinothalamic tract the fibres from the bladder are intermingled with other fibres from the 2nd, 3rd and 4th sacral segments. The same tract conveys impulses that cause strangury, pain in the bladder, pain in the urethra and pain in the lower ureters, vagina and rectum. The same tract conveys impulses causing pleasure in these regions, notably during sexual activity. Many of the fibres in the spinothalamic tracts end around neurons of the reticular formation of the medulla oblongata. Relays of fibres then pass from this region to the centre grey matter of the thalamus. On the medial surface of the cerebral hemisphere in the postcentral and precentral gyri there is a region receiving information from the genitalia and anus, but this does not seem to be a region related to micturition.

SPINAL DAMAGE

From the urological point of view, the level of injury and the degree of completeness are most important. Lesions at a level above the conus medullaris cause flaccid paraplegia and suppress the deep tendon reflexes during the stage of spinal shock. With recovery from spinal shock, hyperreflexia occurs in the deep tendon reflexes below the injury. In these cases acute urinary retention occurs during this phase. It is followed by detrusor hyperreflexia with incontinence upon recovery from the spinal shock. When the spinothalamic tract is divided bilaterally, the patient is not totally deprived of knowledge of the vesical events. He still retains the sensation that micturition is imminent but he notices a new sensation, a vague feeling of fullness which he learns to associate with vesical events. This feeling can be used to tell him when the bladder is full or has just started contracting. The sensation that micturition is imminent is due to afferent impulses from the pelvic and perineal musculature and the urethra. It runs in the sacral part of the posterior column. The feeling that urine is passing comes mainly from the proximal urethra, and most patients with bilateral spinothalamic damage do not feel urine passing. It is, however, a common observation in neurology, that two patients with the same sensory apparatus do not necessarily feel the same sensations.

With injuries to the conus medullaris and cauda equina the deep tendon reflexes are suppressed and there is persistent flaccid weakness associated with urinary retention.

DIAGNOSIS AND ASSESSMENT

Investigations can be designed to help confirm the diagnosis or to assess the urinary tract for complications. The diagnosis is usually obvious from the history and neurological examination. There are, however, three specific physical signs of particular importance in testing for reflex activity of the sacral cord segments:

(1) *Superficial anal reflex.* The skin of the anal margin is pricked with a pin, and a visible contraction of the external anal sphincter is a positive response.

(2) *Bulbocavernous reflex.* This consists of a perineally palpated contraction of the bulbo- and ischiocavernosus muscles in response to squeezing the glans penis or clitoris. This reflex is present in approximately 70 per cent of normal males.

(3) *Ice-water test.* A catheter is passed into the bladder, which is then emptied completely; 60–90 ml of ice-water are instilled, and if the greater part of this is expelled in 60 s, the test is positive.

The first reflexes to appear following spinal cord trauma are usually the bulbocavernosus and superficial anal reflexes. These indicate that there is reflex activity in the sacral segments. This does not mean that there is reflex detrusor activity in response to bladder filling, although it follows that this should eventually occur.

In doubtful cases urodynamic measurements, such as the measure of intravesical pressure, urethral pressure profile and cystometrogram, can be used. Conventional fluid column cystometry has been used for many years to assess patients with neurogenic bladder. This has largely been replaced with modern techniques that give information on the lower urinary tract during filling and voiding. These urodynamic techniques may be combined with electromyographic studies and radiological examination. Other investigations are designed to assess the complications. Regular urine culture from symptomatic and asymptomatic infection and urethral cultures may be required. Measurements of urea, electrolytes and creatinine clearance to assess renal function, intravenous pyelogram for stones and upper tract dilatation, together with a cystogram for reflux and a urethrogram for stricture and diverticulum, are indicated.

TREATMENT OF NEUROGENIC BLADDER

There is no single scheme for treating neurogenic bladder dysfunction. In planning treatment, it is important to consider the underlying disease, the ability of the patient to perform certain manoeuvres with his hands, his ability to reach the bathroom quickly and his ability to co-operate. The aims of treatment should be: (a) preservation of the upper urinary tract, (b) effective control of infection and (c) avoidance of incontinence of urine.

Treatment can be divided into three phases: (1) the acute phase or phase of spinal shock, (2) the re-education phase and (3) the period of definitive treatment.

The acute phase lasts for a few weeks to a few months. During this phase acute retention of urine is normal. Probably the best method of treatment, if the facilities exist and the patient can co-operate, is intermittent catheterisation by the patient. A realistic alternative is an indwelling Foley catheter.

Re-education is a transitional stage when there is a subsidence of spinal shock and progressive appearance of urinary capability and recovery of function of the limbs. During this phase symptoms and objective findings can alter. It is a time when treatment should be expectant, relying on drugs and simple manoeuvres. Definitive procedures should be avoided because functions can be recovered 6 months to 1 year after the acute event. Final treatment is when the patient's clinical condition is stable. The effects on the bladder will depend on the level of injury, as previously discussed, and therefore whether the patient has primary incontinence or retention of urine.

The treatment of neurological incontinence of urine can be difficult. Many types of treatment are available. There are external collecting devices, such as condom urinals, most applicable to male patients. Other methods, such as catheterisation, use of drugs, electrical stimulation and surgical procedures, may also be used in retention of urine, and will be considered in detail later.

It is important to remember that retention can present clinically as overflow incontinence and therefore mimic incontinence. Several methods are available for the treatment of urinary retention. They include abdominal manoeuvres, catheterisation, drugs, neural blocks, electrical stimulation of the bladder and surgical procedures.

Manoeuvres of evacuation

Manoeuvres of evacuation are used exclusively for retention. They consist of: (a) the Credé method, (b) abdominal straining and (c) triggering of bladder function.

The Credé method involves progressive suprapubic compression. Patients with thoracic level lesions have poor abdominal muscles and therefore the Credé method is essential.

Abdominal straining can be used in patients with lumbar lesions, who usually have good diaphragmatic and abdominal muscles. Patients can generate 50–80 cm of water in this way. However, when there is high resistance due to failure of the external sphincter to relax, a surgical procedure on the bladder neck or external sphincter may be required. Before these manoeuvres are started, a cystogram should be performed to see whether vesicoureteric reflux occurs. If present, this contraindicates these procedures because of the risk of causing upper tract deterioration.

Triggering of the bladder is necessary in suprasacral lesions. This is because abdominal strain and the Credé method will induce a reflex contraction of the pelvic floor and a consequent increase of obstruction. Triggering involves any stimulation of the sacral lumbar dermatome and can involve (a) squeezing of the penile area, (b) pulling of pubic hairs, (c) progressive rhythmic suprapubic tapping, (d) digital rectal stimulation and (e) stretching of the external anal sphincter. Frequently these manoeuvres are combined with drugs or surgical procedures. They should be performed by the patient himself or, if incapable, by an attendant. Furthermore, if mobility is a problem, then an external collecting device is also necessary.

Catheterisation

Catheterisation can be used for treating both retention and incontinence. For incontinence it is necessary to have an indwelling catheter. It is usual to use a medium-size 14–16 Foley gauge Silastic-coated catheter which will require changing every 6–8 weeks. The catheter should be inserted with an aseptic technique and a closed drainage system employed. Connection to a leg bag is useful for mobilising patients. Catheter toilet, including cleansing of the urethral meatus, must be practised regularly. Argument persists as to the use of continuous or intermittent drainage. The complications of the latter, such as overdistension with bladder fibrosis, infection and vesicoureteric reflux, outweigh the theoretical advantages. After initial catheterisation most urologists allow rapid decompression of the bladder by free drainage, but although rare, this can be accompanied by bladder haemorrhage. Complications of an indwelling catheter are leakage around the catheter, infection, urethral erosion, diverticula, fistulae and bladder-stones. A most troublesome problem, particularly in females, is leakage around the catheter, sometimes due to the urethra becoming increasingly patulous. Inserting larger-calibre catheters is only ever a short-term solution. It is essential to ensure that the catheter is not blocked. Sometimes, using a retaining balloon of small capacity helps. Giving drugs to prevent bladder spasm may be useful. Infections are better prevented than cured. Other complications are discussed in more detail later. Intermittent self-catheterisation is an ideal that can be achieved in selected patients with retention. Female patients should: (a) wash hands with soap and water, (b) assume lithotomy position with knees apart and (c) insert a well-lubricated 14 Foley gauge catheter.

After initial instruction the patient can perform the procedure while sitting on a toilet-seat. Males can be taught self-catheterisation more easily than females. Catheterisation can be performed in either the sitting or the standing position. Catheters can be prepared for reuse by storing them in detergent or cleaning with soap and water. Catheterisation can be used to manage detrusor areflexia, detrusor hyper-reflexia (when the patient is taking anticholinergic medicine) and detrusor–sphincter dyssynergia.

Pharmacological treatment

Drugs used in the treatment of neurogenic bladder mainly affect the bladder or urethra. When acting on the bladder, they can either increase intravesical pressure and facilitate emptying or suppress bladder contractions and increase capacity. The effect of drugs on the urinary tract is not mediated through a series of receptors, but by two sets of receptors designated α and β.

α *stimulation* is effected by drugs such as phenylephrine, noradrenaline in small doses, choline drugs and some ganglion blockers, such as reserpine. Noradrenaline will increase the bladder pressure when given in small doses and also decreases bladder pressure at the bladder outlet. The α stimulating effect on the urethra is to contract the longitudinal muscles and increase flow resistance. Choline drugs (carbachol, bethanechol, pyridostigmine bromide, distigmine bromide) and α stimulators potentiate each other's actions considerably. The administration of an α stimulating agent greatly increases the urethral pressure.

β *stimulation* results from isoprenaline, adrenaline and noradrenaline in high dosage. They cause relaxation of the detrusor and minimal relaxation of the sphincter.

α *blockade* is effected by Hydergine (co-dergocrine mesylate), phentolamine and phenoxybenzamine. Blockade of α receptors in the detrusor reduces its contractility and is similar to β stimulation in this respect. The urethral adrenergic receptors may be blocked by the drugs noted and the urethral pressure profile falls.

β *blockade* is exemplified by the action of Propranolol. Blockade of the detrusor β receptors reduces the degree to which that muscle can relax. The urethral resistance increases slightly.

The action of drugs on the lower urinary tract is summarised in table 3.1.

Neural blocks can be performed either as diagnostic procedures using Xylocaine or as permanent procedures using phenol block or surgical division. If the procedure is diagnostic, then it should be combined with objective evaluation by cystography and/or pressure measurement.

Table 3.1
Neurogenic bladder: pharmacological treatments

Drugs acting on bladder	Stimulation	Bethanechol chloride Neostigmine bromide Phenoxybenzamine hydrochloride
	Inhibition	Atropine Propantheline bromide Methantheline bromide Oxybutynin Dicyclomine Flavoxate (Urispas) Imipramine (Tofranil)
Drugs acting on bladder neck and urethra	Stimulation	Ephedrine sulphate Imipramine (Tofranil) Ornade (with phenylpropanolamine)
	Inhibition	Phenoxybenzamine Methyldopa (Aldomet)

Pudendal neurectomy can be effective but is associated with impotence in 50–60 per cent of cases. It may also cause anaesthesia in the perivaginal and perianal region, and bowel incontinence. Sacral block transforms a hyperreflexic bladder into an areflexic one. It carries a high risk of impotence and bowel incontinence. Furthermore, the areflexic bladder then requires manoeuvres to empty it.

Surgical procedures

Transurethral resection of the bladder neck (TUR) will decrease resistance of bladder neck in retention.

External sphincterotomy (figures 3.1, 3.2) is now commonly used, employing either a cutting Collins knife or a transurethral resection loop. Possible complications are profuse bleeding due to the spongy tissue of the penis being entered, extravasation of urine and sepsis. Urethral strictures can occur as a late complication. The success rate is high, and upper urinary tract dilatation, vesicoureteric reflux, residual urine and recurrence of urinary tract infection can be reduced. However, total destruction of the sphincter will cause incontinence and then an external collecting device is necessary. Sometimes the combination of a more judicious sphincterotomy with evacuation manoeuvres will result in an acceptable degree of continence.

Operations to reduce bladder capacity. A primarily enlarged bladder is rarely a problem and it is usually secondary to outflow obstruction. Obstruction must therefore be dealt with first, and if volume reduction is necessary, it can be achieved by excision or imbrication of the bladder wall.

Operation to increase bladder capacity involves ileocystoplasty or caecoplasty. Although cystoplasty may increase bladder capacity, the sphincter is frequently affected, which leads to incontinence. Careful preoperative assessment is therefore essential.

Urinary diversion: (a) perineal urethrostomy, (b) cystotomy, (c) anterior urethral diversion and (d) supravesical diversion.

Cystotomy involves marsupialisation of the bladder to the

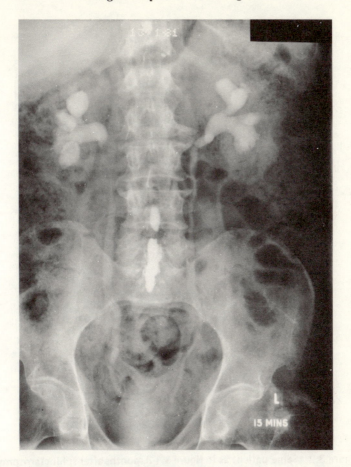

Figure 3.1 Intravenous pyelogram showing dilatation of the ureters, renal pelvis and calyces before treatment.

anterior wall of the abdomen, with an appropriate collecting device. Continent cystotomy can be performed, but intermittent self-catheterisation is then required through a constructed tube from the bladder to the abdominal wall. This intermittent catheterisation carries the same risk as urethral catheterisation. It is not commonly performed in females, where the same effect can be achieved by transposing the urethra to the anterior abdominal wall. Cystotomy may be

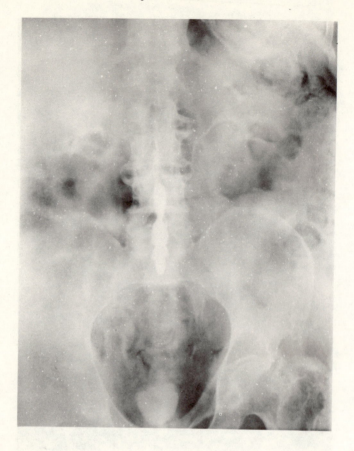

Figure 3.2   Same patient as in figure 3.1 3 months after sphincterotomy.

useful to rid those patients with continuing sexual ability of indwelling urethral catheters. Cystotomy may be combined with ligation of the urethra.

Supravesical diversion into an ileal or colonic loop is indicated in 1–3 per cent of patients when progressive upper tract dilatation occurs due to either destruction by a hyperactive bladder or intractable vesicoureteric reflux. Ureterosigmoid anastomosis is usually contraindicated because of the poor bowel control in most patients.

Electronic control of the micturition reflex

These methods include: (a) stimulation of the spinal cord, (b) stimulation of the pelvic nerve innervation of the detrusor muscle, (c) stimulation of one or more sacral ventral roots innervating the detrusor muscle, (d) direct application of electrodes to the detrusor muscle, and (e) stimulation of periurethral striated muscles for incontinence.

No stimulation site has overwhelming superiority. Pain, spread of the stimulus and alteration of the neuromuscular excitability are major disadvantages of these methods. Stimulation of the urethra is achieved by either an anal plug and external stimulation or implanted electrodes with a subcutaneous receiver stimulator. Infection and broken electrodes can also be a problem with these.

Artificial urinary sphincters

The requirements of the artificial sphincter are: (a) total implantability, (b) construction materials compatible with body tissues, (c) high enough pressure to provide continence but not so high as to affect urethral viability, and (d) pressure release that allows rises of intravesical pressure without injuring the upper tracts.

One such device is shown in figure 3.3. Although the concept is attractive, only limited success can be achieved at present. Infection of the implant and mechanical failure are common problems.

COMPLICATIONS OF NEUROGENIC BLADDER

Complications of neurogenic bladder include: (a) stone formation, (b) vesicoureteric reflux, (c) urethral diverticula and fistulae, (d) urethral stenosis and (e) urinary tract infection.

Stone formation occurs in 10–15 per cent of patients with neurogenic bladder. The bladder (figure 3.4) is the commonest site, but stones also occur in the kidneys and ureters (figure 3.5). They are predisposed to by poor urinary tract drainage,

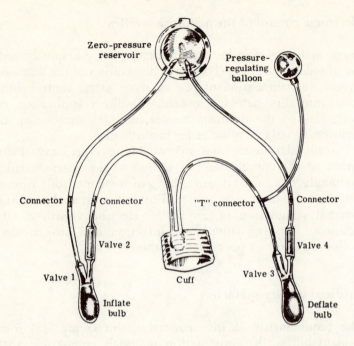

Figure 3.3 An artificial urinary sphincter using a compression cuff
Model AS761 (after Raz and Bradley, 1979).

urinary infection, hypercalcuria due to immobilisation and
encrustation of urinary catheters. Treatment is by usual
surgical principles. In the bladder, stones can be crushed by
lithotrite and then washed out. Large stones, very hard stones
or complicating pathology may necessitate suprapubic
removal. Stones in the upper tracts require removal if they
are causing obstruction, persistent infection or pain, or if
they are enlarging rapidly. Once they have been treated
surgically, prophylactic treatment should be started to
prevent recurrence. This includes high fluid intake, possibly
combined with a thiazide diuretic and correction of predisposing factors.

Vesicoureteric reflux occurs in 10–40 per cent of patients,
but is usually secondary to poor bladder drainage. Correction
of outflow obstruction by surgery or catheterisation will

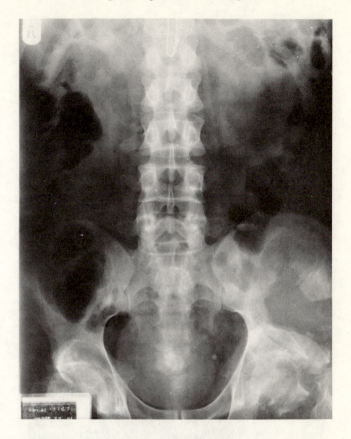

Figure 3.4   Abdominal X-ray to show multiple bladder stones.

usually improve reflux. Antireflux operations may be indicated for persisting reflux and even supravesical urinary diversion may be required in persistent cases.

Urethral diverticula and fistulae mainly occur in the male, and result from urethral catheters, external collecting devices or penile clamps. Urinary diversion, urethroplasty and antibiotics may be needed. Urethral strictures result from similar causes, with the addition of traumatic instrumentation. Treatment by dilatation, urethrotomy or urethroplasty is indicated.

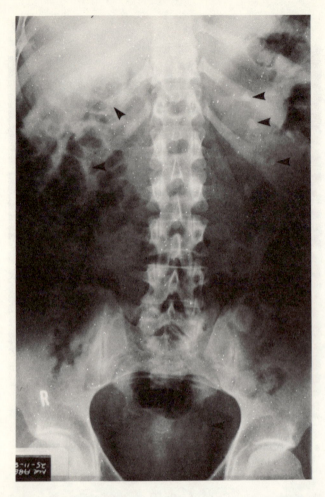

Figure 3.5 Abdominal X-ray to show multiple stones in both kidneys and ureters. Subsequently removed surgically.

Urinary tract infections are the most common complications of neurogenic bladder. They result from urinary stasis, poor hydration, anatomical abnormality, stones and catheterisation. Prevention is better than cure. Correction of predisposing causes is essential. Prophylactic antibiotics are not indicated, as they encourage resistant organisms to occur.

Bladder irrigation with an antiseptic, such as 1:5000 aqueous Hibitane or Noxyflex, may be useful in those patients with indwelling urethral catheters. Treatment of symptomatic cases and those with systemic infections with appropriate antibiotics indicated by urinary culture is essential.

SEXUAL FUNCTION

In men with complete motor neuron lesions, spontaneous or reflex erections occur frequently and 70 per cent are able to have coitus, although the majority cannot ejaculate or experience orgasm. Eighty per cent of men with incomplete upper motor neuron lesions are capable of erection and coitus. Those with less extensive upper motor neuron lesions are more likely to ejaculate. In contrast, 75 per cent of men with lower motor neuron injuries are impotent. The remaining 25 per cent are capable of psychogenic erection; but even in some of these, erection was too short for coitus, and only a few of them could ejaculate.

PROGNOSIS

Careful follow-up of spinal cord injury patients has given much useful information regarding the importance of the urological complications. In one series of 1851 patients with traumatic paraplegia, studied between 1946 and 1965, the commonest cause of later death was renal failure, which occurred in 32.9 per cent. Death from renal failure is more common in patients with damage at the thoracic level.

In another study patients were divided into those with good bladder function (characterised by no ureteric reflux and a residual urine of less than one-third of the bladder capacity) and poor bladder function. Twenty per cent of those with poor bladder function survived 25 years, whereas 50 per cent of the good group were alive and the majority of deaths were due to renal disease.

Such data emphasise the importance of the careful management of the urinary tract in patients with neurological disease.

BIBLIOGRAPHY

Band, D. (1963). *Spinal Injuries*, Morrison and Gibb, Edinburgh.

Bors, E. (1957). Neurogenic bladder. *Urol. Surv.*, 1, 177–250.

Bors, E. and Comars, A. E. (1971). *Neurological Urology*, University Park Press, Baltimore.

Eckstein, H. B. (1974). Neuropathic bladder. In *Urology in Childhood* (Ed. L. Williams), Springer-Verlag, New York.

Gibbon, N. (1966). Management of the bladder in acute and chronic disorders of the nervous system. *Acta neurol. scand.*, 42, 133.

Gibbon, N. O. K. (1976). Later management of the paraplegic bladder. *Paraplegia*, 12, 87.

Pearman, J. W. and England, E. J. (1973). *The Urological Management of the Patient following Spinal Cord Injury*, Charles C. Thomas, Springfield, Ill.

Raz, S. and Bradley, W. E. (1979). *Urology*, Vol. 2. (Eds J. H. Harrison, R. F. Gittes, A. D. Perlmutter, T. A. Stamey and P. C. Walsh), Saunders, London and Toronto, Chapter 35, 1215–1270.

Scott, F. B., Bradley, W. N. and Timm, G. W. (1974). Treatment of urinary incontinence by an implantable prosthetic sphincter. *J. Urol.*, 112, 75.

4. The role of the physiotherapist

Ida Bromley

When a perfectly healthy robust person is changed in a few seconds into one who is totally dependent as a result of acute paraplegia, he is frightened and lost in a strange world. He cannot move or feel his limbs, and has no bladder, bowel or sexual function. In addition, other injuries may be present. This human being, dependent upon others for all normal physical functions, has to become what Sir Ludwig Guttmann termed a 'spinal man' (Guttmann, 1973).

The physical aspect of rehabilitation embraces the various components shown in figure 4.1. The physiotherapist, working with other members of the rehabilitation team involved in this metamorphosis from dependent human being to independent 'spinal man', is predominantly concerned with movement.

When patients with paraplegia were first gathered together at Stoke Mandeville Hospital under the care of Sir Ludwig Guttmann in 1944, only one physiotherapist at the hospital could be persuaded to undertake work in the new Spinal Unit. The only physiotherapy known for such patients at that time was entirely 'passive', consisting of passive movements to the limbs while the patient died from pressure sores and/or renal failure. As is well known, Sir Ludwig Guttmann soon changed that image by teaching physiotherapists to rehabilitate function, until there was a queue of physiotherapists from all parts of the world waiting to work in his unit.

The role of the physiotherapist will be examined in terms of clinical practice, secondary prevention, home care and the rehabilitation team.

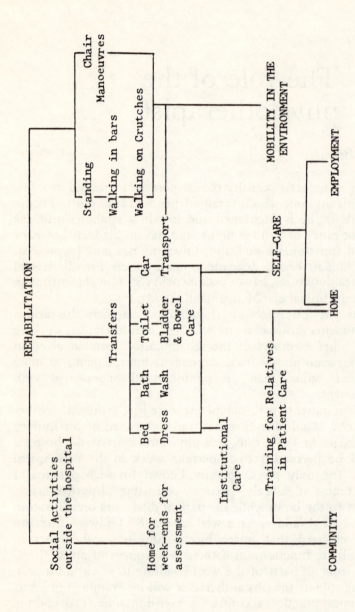

Figure 4.1 Progress from dependent human being to independent 'spinal man'.

CLINICAL PRACTICE

The physiotherapist's role in teaching the paraplegic patient how to move again, how to lift his paralysed limbs, how to transfer, walk and manoeuvre in the environment, has been quite clearly defined for a long time. However, certain changes have occurred in the treatment of paraplegia and in the approach of physiotherapists to their work in this field.

Correct early positioning of patients with spinal cord injury has always been emphasised in order to prevent contractures and to minimise the development of extreme spasticity. As knowledge of the effect of posture on spasticity has increased, so there have been changes in the way patients are positioned in bed in the early weeks following injury. For example, when the paraplegic patient is supine, the legs are usually placed in extension. However, if extensor spasticity is extreme, flexion of the hips and knees may be desirable in order to inhibit the predominant extensor synergy. Similarly, particularly when the lesion is incomplete and spasticity often severe, the supine position may only be used infrequently, the side lying position being used for the greater part of the 24 hours. Little is known about the input, if any, to the central nervous system during the period of spinal shock. Greater knowledge in this field might further affect the attitude to and practice of early positioning.

Physiotherapists, with their interest in spasticity, have been urging the changes described above. The bilateral approach to the rehabilitation of patients with brain damage, as advocated by Mrs Bertha Bobath, has become popular with physiotherapists treating patients with neurological deficit resulting from injury to the spinal cord, where that injury has resulted in an incomplete cord lesion above the cauda equina level.

Mrs Bobath, in the second edition of her book *Adult Hemiplegia* (Bobath, 1978), states: 'The aim of this treatment is to help the patient to gain control over the patterns of spasticity by inhibiting the abnormal reflex patterns. This process of inhibition is combined with special techniques of handling the patient so as to "facilitate" the movement patterns of the higher integrated righting and equilibrium reactions, for example, the static-kinetic movement patterns of the normal postural reflex mechanism, which allow for normal functional activity.' The problem for physiotherapists treating paraplegic patients with incomplete cord lesions has always been that of realising the potential of the patients' active movement when hampered by severe spasticity. Mrs Bobath's approach is proving invaluable in the treatment of such patients.

A new approach to treatment using the Gymnastic Ball has recently been introduced to physiotherapists in this country by Domenica Hasler. This treatment, originally devised by Dr S. Klein-Vogelbach in Switzerland, involves the use of large balls of different diameters. While the ball is used in various ways as a support, exercises are given to retrain equilibrium reactions, increase strength, reduce spasticity and initiate functional activity for any part of the body. Again, this type of treatment is particularly valuable for patients with incomplete lesions, although it is also used to reduce spasticity for patients with complete lesions.

Some recently developed biofeedback devices are proving of help in physiotherapy rehabilitation programmes. One example is the pressure device used under wheelchair cushions in the form of an alarm bell. The bell rings if the patient does not relieve the weight off his ischial tuberosities within a 10 min period. This device can perhaps help the more forgetful patient to become effectively pressure-conscious. Fairly simple, though not inexpensive, biofeedback machines are now obtainable which can assist in muscle development by showing the patient his rate of achievement and progress, and, incidentally, by necessitating the setting of objectives.

Changes have occurred in recent years in the 'hardware' used by the paraplegic patient which may or may not be deemed 'progress', according to the viewpoint of the therapist. One undoubted area of advance has been in wheelchair design. Although total satisfaction has not yet been achieved, the wheelchair has nevertheless been streamlined in comparison with the large, rigid, brown leather upholstered wheelchairs used at Stoke Mandeville in the early days.

The recent addition of the kerb climber to some wheelchairs facilitates movement in the environment for those who find it difficult to push the chair unaided up a kerb. The wheelchair, which converts from the seated to the standing position, now brings otherwise impossible daily tasks within the scope of the paraplegic patient. One paraplegic physiotherapist finds such a chair an essential piece of equipment in his daily practice in the wards and department of a district general hospital.

Although for many years, both in and outside spinal units, therapists have been sharing their knowledge with the medical profession when ordering wheelchairs for their patients, they are now preparing to accept the responsibility, which assuredly will be theirs in the future, for prescribing models of wheelchairs.

Attempts have been made over the past few years to improve the calipers used by paraplegic patients. The Pneumatic Support Garment, the Swivel Walker and the Hip Guidance Orthosis are all being used by some patients in the UK, although none to date has received universal acclaim.

Physiotherapists around the world have progressed over the past few years to a more realistic approach in their expectations of teaching the paraplegic patient with a complete lesion to walk with calipers and crutches. Until recently all paraplegic patients with lesions at T5 and below were expected to learn to walk in this way. Several research papers have been written recently showing that fewer than 50 per cent of patients use their calipers to walk after leaving hospital when their initial period of rehabilitation is completed (Mikelberg, 1981). Even the superior caliper developed at the Craig Rehabilitation Centre, Colorado, USA, produced no higher results. Only 8 per cent used the calipers for total functional use, although this study emphasised the psychological importance to the patient of learning to walk even if the patient chose not to continue to do so (O'Daniel, 1981).

Perhaps these results are not surprising, considering some of the other research which has been carried out in the last few years in relation to the high energy cost involved in walking with crutches.

Since its introduction in 1944 sport has played a part in the rehabilitation of paralysed patients. Over the years the International Games for the Paralysed, first introduced at

Stoke Mandeville, grew and developed into the International Games for the Paralysed and Other Disabled. These games are now held annually for each disability group. Every four years these groups combine to hold the Olympics for the Disabled. These coincide with the able-bodied Olympics and are often held in the same country.

CLINICAL SCIENCE

Clinical science incorporates research and education as well as clinical practice.

Physiotherapy in the treatment of paraplegia encompasses an extensive and impressive area of clinical practice. Attempts to scrutinise the science behind these procedures are few, perhaps because, to date, the measurable components in rehabilitation are also few. However, progress is being made, for physiotherapists are now speculating about their practice and discussion on the 'art versus science' theme can be heard in all branches of the profession. Time is beginning to play an important part in the physiotherapist's thinking in relation to the rehabilitation programme. How can the physiotherapist more speedily develop and retrain the 'bridge muscles' joining the paralysed and non-paralysed areas of the body and the new balance reactions used so extensively by spinal man, so that the patient spends less of his life in hospital? What causes the difference between the successful and unsuccessful groups of patients in rehabilitation? Is it the one-to-one relationship with the patient – the therapist–patient interaction – that makes the difference? The intangible link between patient and therapist results in the patient gaining confidence in the therapist and establishes their mutual identification with a common objective. Basmajian (1975) stated: 'When one views the whole field of rehabilitation including physiotherapy one is struck by the impression that rehabilitation's main virtue is *not* its scientific base. Rather its main virtue is the intensive relationship of the various professionals with individual patients.'

Is there a need to identify predictive factors to help the workers in this field to differentiate between those who will be successful in their overall rehabilitation programme and those who will not — those, for example, who will use their calipers after leaving hospital? Some work has been done on this aspect in relation to tetraplegia. In such cases, where the period of hospitalisation is so much longer, there is an even greater need to avoid extra weeks spent trying to learn to perform activities which will not be put to use in daily living at home. Most therapists would agree that every effort should be made to help each patient achieve his optimum perform-ance, but there would appear to be less support for the opposite view that it is detrimental to the patient to be given expectations which cannot be realised.

Research

Research is constantly being undertaken in the specialist medical and surgical fields related to paraplegia. Its only bearing, if implemented, on physiotherapy is to make the patient fitter and more able to be active. The results of recent and continuing research in neuroanatomy may help to provide a scientific basis for techniques which physio-therapists have used and found effective for years. The number of physiotherapists involved in research is minimal. The major progress to date, certainly in England, is the therapists' change in attitude towards research. As always, progress is slow. This is hardly surprising, as it is only recently that physiotherapists have begun to think critically and to speculate about what they are doing and how they are doing it.

Education

In the endeavour to marry art and science in physiotherapy, some thought needs to be given to education and to the way post-registration education is carried out. In 1975 Licht, after observing physiotherapy techniques in the neurosciences, stated: 'Techniques are passed on from therapist to therapist by demonstration — often with the mystique associated with

Ida Bromley

a religious ritual.' This is certainly true of the treatment of paraplegia. In this exchange of information the major emphasis is often placed on the performance of the technique, and there is therefore a tendency to justify practice on the basis of personal observation. Teaching and learning can become almost entirely a technical event with little concern for the underlying physiological and pathological processes.

SECONDARY PREVENTION

While the patient is in hospital, it is hoped that complications will be avoided or satisfactorily resolved. However, when the patient is finally discharged home at the end of the initial period of rehabilitation, there is often no further contact with a physiotherapist. Although the spinal units recall their patients for periodic checks, few patients see the physiotherapist at that time. Yet the physiotherapist certainly has a role in relation to the prevention of further handicap. For a variety of reasons patients sometimes develop a bad posture in the wheelchair, with resultant problems, such as an increase in spasticity, which can give rise to pressure sores or to contractures. If these become serious, day-to-day function can become affected. The patient may no longer be able to sit comfortably in the wheelchair or transfer independently and thus may be unable to go out of the home.

The *International Classification of Impairments, Disabilities and Handicaps*, published by the World Health Organisation in 1980, must prove to be a great help to all those involved in the care of patients with disabling diseases, including physiotherapists working with paraplegic patients. This classification, developed by Dr Philip Wood and others, is described as 'a manual of classification relating to the consequence of disease'.

$$\left.\begin{array}{l} \text{injury} \\ \text{disease} \end{array}\right\} \text{impairment} - \text{disability} - \text{handicap}$$

Disease or injury produces *impairment* — that is, some abnormality of body structure or appearance. As a result of the impairment, the 'performance' or 'behaviour' of the individual may be altered. This is described as *disability*. *Disability* occurs in terms of functional performance and activity by the individual. This altered behaviour or performance may place the individual at a disadvantage relative to other people. The disadvantage limits or prevents the fulfilment of a role that is normal for that individual in comparison with his peers. This disadvantage at the social level is termed *handicap*.

This classification will surely help to identify which of the patient's problems result purely from his original impairment and which arise as a result of neglect which could possibly have been prevented.

Clinical example 1

Scoliosis is a common problem. The power in the trunk muscles of a paraplegic patient with an injury at T12 may be of unequal strength on each side of the body, so that the patient develops a long 'C' curvature of the spine to one side, usually to the side of the dominant hand. As a result, some muscles will become contracted while others are overstretched. Distortion of the spine and pelvis through habitual abnormal posture results. Increased spasticity resulting in poor balance may follow, and, in extreme cases, loss of independence in transfers, particularly to cars.

Clinical example 2

A patient with a lower thoracic lesion, who is able to walk with calipers, may be unable to walk for a while, possibly because of a pressure sore or some renal problem. The hip flexors may become contracted and the patient no longer has the extreme flexibility of the hip joints necessary to walk well with calipers and crutches. This may be relatively unimportant for some patients, but for others it may mean the difference between being totally independent at an airport or in a hotel and being unable to travel without assistance.

In each of these examples the patient's resultant handicap in society is increased, whereas caught early enough the handicap could probably have been prevented.

HOME CARE

For a long time there have been pleas from those working in spinal units to have a system of home care for patients subsequent to discharge. The Spinal Unit at the Robert Jones and Agnes Hunt Orthopaedic Hospital in Oswestry has led the field in this direction in relation to the nursing and overall care of the patient. Physiotherapists in other units are making greater endeavours to see at least all patients with incomplete lesions during their follow-up examinations. The developments in physiotherapy community services and the expanding facilities for general practitioners to refer patients to local physiotherapy services now make provision for patients with spinal cord injury or disease to receive care at home as and when they need it.

The DHSS publication circulated from the Department of Health and Social Security entitled (1) *Physiotherapy in the Community* and (2) *Open Access for General Practitioners* provides support for those district therapists anxious to set up these services. The blurring of the boundary between hospital and home also allows specialist physiotherapists from the hospital to visit patients with particular problems in their homes and, should it be necessary, to arrange further treatment in the hospital physiotherapy department.

Some departments now keep an 'at risk' register of patients with permanent disability, including those with paralysis resulting from spinal cord injury or disease, and the therapist sees them as appropriate. Patients, though aware that their situation is deteriorating, are often loath to return to their spinal unit unless the problem is acute. For many, to visit the spinal unit means a considerable journey and may also mean loss of time at work. An apparently minor problem may progress to such an extent that handicap is all too often increased before treatment is obtained — so *observation + action = prevention.*

Today the developing systems of community care can aid prevention. However, it is questionable whether physiotherapists in a local department would know what to do even if they recognised the problem. Why is it that so little has been achieved in nearly 40 years in the education of the members of the various professions who work in general hospitals about the treatment of the paraplegic, let alone the tetraplegic patient?

THE REHABILITATION TEAM

In recent years much has been written about the multidisciplinary team approach to patient care. Two main reasons exist for its mention here.

First, to reinstate and to stress the extreme importance to the patient of being at the centre of a team of people who share their knowledge and speak with a united voice (Bromley, 1981). The atmosphere of hope and confidence which they create around the patient enables lost self-confidence to be recovered and maximum benefit to be gained from the rehabilitation programme. The physiotherapist in such a team shares in creating the right atmosphere and carrying out unit policies. Where there is no team approach, the result for the patient is confusion, fear and depression. Inevitably this has a marked effect on the patient's response to physiotherapy, and rehabilitation is slow, if indeed it is ever successful.

The second reason is to raise a question. In the last 10 years has any progress been made in the treatment of those paraplegic patients who never reach the spinal units? From time to time these patients are found in orthopaedic, neurological, neurosurgical and general medical wards of district general hospitals. Until there are many more spinal units built in the UK, not all paraplegic patients will be able to be transferred to spinal units in the foreseeable future. Even if, in the general hospital, one member of the multidisciplinary team is knowledgeable about the treatment of paraplegia, this is not sufficient to provide either adequate treatment or the atmosphere of confidence so necessary to the patients' welfare.

Would it not be possible to have a small team — a doctor, a nurse and a physiotherapist — in each health district who would be willing at least to learn the *rudiments* of care for these patients and could take on their management? The general principles of treatment are not difficult to learn, or to put into practice, where there is enthusiasm for the care of patients with this problem.

If we have any doubts that the patients with paraplegia admitted to district general hospitals in 1990 will receive more expert management than they do today, we should plan now to ensure that the doubt is unfounded.

REFERENCES

Basmajian, J. V. (1975). Research or retrench. *Phys. Ther. J.*, 55, 607–610.

Bobath, B. (1978). *Adult Hemiplegia*, 2nd edn, Heinemann, London.

Bromley, A. I. (1981). *Tetraplegia and Paraplegia: A Guide for Physiotherapists*, 2nd edn, Churchill Livingstone, Edinburgh.

Guttmann, Sir L. (1973). *Spinal Cord Injuries: Comprehensive Management and Research*, Blackwell, London.

Licht, S. (1975). In *Stroke and its Rehabilitation*, New Haven, Conn.

Mikelberg, R. (1981). Spinal cord lesions and lower extremity bracing: An overview and follow-up study. *Paraplegia*, 379–385.

O'Daniel, W. E. (1981). Follow-up usage of the Scott–Craig orthosis in paraplegia. *Paraplegia*, 19, 373–378.

World Health Organisation (1980). *International Classification of Impairments, Disabilities and Handicaps*, Geneva.

5. The role of the occupational therapist

Gill Arnott

Paraplegia, by virtue of its less devastating physical disabilities, would, at first appearance, seem to require less in the way of occupational therapy than the more severely disabled tetraplegic patient. It is all too easy to fall into the habit of referring to 'John Smith having sustained only a paraplegia', whereas to John Smith his paraplegic disability is total devastation and apparent loss of everything previously known.

Occupational therapy within the rehabilitation team has an increasingly important part to play in the successful retraining in physical independence and social rehabilitation of the paraplegic patient. Because of their dual physical/psychological qualifications and training, occupational therapists are well equipped to adapt and adjust to the varying requirements, personalities and needs of these individuals, ranging from young trendy motor-cyclists to older, steadier yet determined characters who make up the varied and interesting case load.

PERSONAL INDEPENDENCE

Treatment is aimed at achieving maximum personal independence in the following ways:

Maximum strength in the innervated muscles of upper limbs and trunk.

An improvement of balance, posture and co-ordination.

An awareness of the difficulties associated with loss of sensation, with practical advice for safe management in this respect.

Successful home resettlement if at all possible, with advice on alterations, aids and adaptations, with support and advice to relatives.

The provision of information and advice on mobility and such help as the conversion of cars to hand controls.

Job resettlement and re-employment possibilities.

Social confidence and awareness, and help in psychological development of personalities to assist in overcoming disability and its related problems.

Ideas and opportunities for the development of hobbies/leisure/sporting activities.

An information and advice service for all aspects of rehabilitation, resettlement, attainments and pleasure in a patient's future life.

These aims to personal independence are considered in more detail under the following headings: dressing, transfer and homecraft.

Paraplegics have normal function of their upper limbs, and independence retraining is therefore primarily guided towards activities requiring management of their paralysed, seemingly heavy, immobile and useless lower limbs.

Dressing

Initial practice for dressing is commenced on the bed, as this provides a wide and relatively safe working base. Early difficulties may include poor balance, lack of confidence and inability to sit up from a lying position. With reassurance, guidance and encouragement most paraplegics quickly attain this independence. Occupational therapists teach one of a series of 'known' and tried methods, but always encourage patients to develop and practise their own variations.

(1) The patient sits up in bed with the legs extended. Garments are slipped over the feet by using trunk flexion and extended arms to reach the feet. The clothes are then pulled up the legs to mid-thigh level or higher. The patient lies flat, and by rolling from side to side can reach to pull pants and trousers in turn up over the buttocks.

(2) The patient sits up in bed supported by pillows against the backrest. In this method the arms are used to pull up or lift the legs in turn towards the chest so that garments may be slipped over the appropriate foot and then be moved up the legs. Lying flat and using the rolling technique is again practised for pulling the clothes up further.

(3) Patients with incomplete spinal lesions may find it easier to dress sitting over the side of the bed.

(4) Practice is often extended eventually to include dressing in the wheelchair. This is sometimes more appropriate and easy to fit into a routine at home — for example, after using the toilet or bath — and may also be more applicable later when the patient attends local swimming baths, where changing rooms are often inaccessible or unsuitable.

(5) Advice is given on the application and fitting of any urinary devices worn, and the patient is encouraged to check the position of the drainage tube after dressing and any transfer.

Use of aids

Actual aids are seldom used when dressing, as a change of technique normally overcomes any difficulties and insensitive skin demands extra care from scratches and abrasions, but the following may prove useful. Care must also always be taken that 'aids', if used, are not left loose in the bed.

A firm orthopaedic-type mattress.

A monkey pole or lifting handle at the bedhead helps with manoeuvres and transfers.

Use of a long reacher, wrap-around skirts for ladies and zips inserted into inside trouser leg seams may be useful additions. Advice should be given on recommended clothing, materials, styles and sizes.

A therapist's attitude during dressing practice must be practical, confident and reassuring.

Lack of success in independent dressing can result from the following: continued poor balance; a large body build; the presence of sharp spinal or rib pain, particularly on trunk flexion; increased spasticity of the lower limbs; overpossessive relatives who are too eager to provide unnecessary assistance; a lack of persistence or interest on the part of the patient, for whom dressing is a challenge which initially requires effort and energy.

Transfers

Transfers are ideally taught by all members of the rehabilitation team and included as appropriate during a patient's daily routine. Great care must be taken to perfect good strong transfers which eliminate the danger of abrasion or other damage to insensitive areas. Most paraplegics ultimately require little in the way of assistance or aids for transferring, although temporary aids may be needed until strength and confidence increase.

Methods of transfer are as follows.

Wheelchair to bed

(a) Sideways with chair arm removed and wheel protectively covered. Legs are lifted on to the bed first, with the rest of the body following through.

(b) The chair, with footplates swung back out of the way, is placed at right angles to the bed for a forward/backward transfer on to and off the bed.

Wheelchair to WC

(a) Sideways transfer is the easiest and most efficient transfer to be taught initially. The wheel should be protectively covered and brakes firmly applied.

(b) Forward transfer, with the chair at a slight angle to the WC, by a lifting swinging movement.

(c) Forward transfer, directly on to WC with the paraplegic facing the wall.

(d) For some a backward approach through a zipped chair-back canvas may be a solution. Forward transfer back on to the chair can be a difficulty with this technique.

Aids for toilet transfers include:

A raised toilet seat to bring a low WC up to wheelchair seat height.

Protective inflatable rubber toilet seat cover.

Wall rail.

Non-slip flooring strips.

It is always useful to discover which method of transfer is easiest for a patient and to practise this, but it must be applied to the actual transfer which will be required at home. Care must also be taken to ensure that, before discharge, a patient has practised a variety of approaches and transfers on to WCs. This is particularly important for women, who when bladder-trained require access to a toilet every 3–4 h. In a friend's house, or public place, facilities may be limited and totally different from those with which they are familiar. The confidence gained through the ability to transfer by varying methods ensures success.

Wheelchair to bath

This transfer must, again, be practised in relation to what will be required at home, unless a purpose-built unit is planned. Getting into the bath normally presents minimum difficulty, but for many getting out of the bath and on to the wheelchair poses a major problem. The following methods are taught:

(a) A sideways transfer, with wheel protected, is the usual method suitable for use in most bathrooms. The legs are lifted into the bath first, with the rest of the body following through. The lift back out of the bath requires strength control, and many find it necessary to rest on the back bath-sill before completing the transfer back into the wheel-chair.

(b) Where possible and where space permits, it is often easier to transfer in over the end of the bath, where the sloping back of the bath provides a useful slide for the transfer back up into the chair.

Useful aids for the bathroom include:

An over-bathboard at the back of the bath can extend the 'resting area'. In some bathrooms it may be possible to provide this same facility behind the bath in the form of a Formica bench or shelf.

Non-slip bath-mat.

Ideally water should be released from the bath before the transfer out occurs, and the patient encouraged to dry off excess water. Some patients find, however, that the buoyancy and 'lift' provided by the bath-water does facilitate this transfer.

Half-way bath-seat from which the patient can either bathe or use a shower attachment from the taps and yet independently transfer back out from the bath.

Showers are becoming increasingly popular and more accepted by society generally. A paraplegic can easily transfer on to a suitable shower-chair, and with the tap for a thermostatically controlled shower within reach may complete the shower independently, safely and with ease.

Wheelchair to car

(a) *As a passenger.* Initially this transfer is greatly assisted by the use of a transfer or sliding board until strength and confidence increase. The legs are placed into the well of the car first with the rest of the body following. On the reverse transfer the legs remain in the car until last.

(b) *As a driver.* A driver may wish independently to load the wheelchair into the car back-seat space. The easiest method of teaching this is for the patient to transfer initially into the passenger-seat of the car. The footplates can then be removed from the wheelchair and the chair-back dropped if possible. The chair is folded up and positioned at right angles to the car, against, or resting on, the sill, in line with the back-seat space. The patient transfers into the driving-seat. The front passenger-seat can be lifted forward, and by reaching behind this, the chair can be grasped and pulled into the back of the car. Some paraplegics prefer to transfer direct into the driver's seat by preparing the chair, transferring their bottom only on to the passenger-seat so that the driver's seat can then be lifted forward and the wheelchair loaded into the car, before returning to the driving position.

Useful aids for drivers include:

Transfer board made of timber smoothly sanded and polished or varnished to provide a sliding surface.

A less expensive board can be made from plywood and protectively covered with Fablon or contact material. The length and width of the board can be individually determined, but a standard board measures 2 ft 6 in (778 mm) × 8 in (203 mm), with rounded ends.

Wheelchair to easy chair

Many paraplegics prefer a change of position and seating. Transferring into a soft, cushioned chair presents little difficulty, but the return transfer is usually 'uphill', with little in the way of a firm surface available to assist with the necessary 'push up'. The easiest ways of overcoming this problem are:

To insert a wooden board under the easychair cushion to increase firmness.

To add a second cushion to the easychair to increase its height.

To raise the whole chair with special blocks.

To remove the wheelchair cushion before the transfer back so that height difference is reduced. The cushion should be replaced immediately afterwards.

Homecraft

Kitchen work

Women and men paraplegics should be encouraged to participate in kitchen activities, so that on discharge they can confidently and safely prepare anything from a hot drink, cakes or snacks, to a full meal. Attention is paid to the home kitchen layout and practice or advice given where appropriate. Common-sense is required to reposition the contents of a kitchen cupboard so that the heaviest or most often used items become the most easily accessible. Many paraplegics find the use of a wheelchair table beneficial, so that not only do they have an ideal working surface at all times, but also they are not tempted to use their lap as a carrying surface. Advance meal planning and preparation, together with efficient use of modern appliances such as multi-mixers, coffee filters, freezers, mini-grills or microwave ovens, facilitate independence in the kitchen.

Housework

Most paraplegics can manage basic and routine jobs around the house, given reasonable access to all rooms, but for heavier chores the services of home helps or relatives are often much appreciated.

Continental quilts assist bed-making; built-in bedroom furniture and careful positioning of other household furniture can provide easier access; while the removal of loose mats or rugs can greatly improve mobility around the house.

Laundry

Within the department there are usually facilities for patients to attend to their own washing and ironing requirements, which encourages independence in laundry management.

UPPER LIMB AND TRUNK STRENGTHENING

Activity in the occupational therapy workshop can be used to develop maximum strength and co-ordination of innervated muscles. Upper limb strength is of paramount importance to give independence to paraplegics through good transfers and activity generally. With careful grading and planning, and given encouragement, paraplegics can be progressed from fairly uncomplicated satisfying activities introducing them to 'working from a wheelchair' to activities presenting a challenge, and requiring strength, dexterity and balance.

Many of today's young people do not conform to this ideal, refusing to do anything remotely resembling hard work. To force the issue at the time would only cause antagonism and result in their total absence from the department, which would lead to their missing all the support and advice that can subsequently be given. As therapists, we learn to be more subtle in our approach and to use a wide range of different yet interesting and attractive activities, while still fulfilling the basic criteria in our aims of treatment.

Clinical example

It is not uncommon for a young male paraplegic to view woodwork or metal work with reluctance and disinterest. It would be more sensible to anticipate this reaction and in its place suggest a game of table football or pool. These would involve balance, co-ordination, bilateral activity, dexterity, concentration, enjoyment, and a sense of participation and competition which fulfil the aims of treatment, together with development of social skills and confidence.

It is not unusual for the patient then to progress voluntarily to other activity, such as woodwork and metal work.

The following activities are valuable in strengthening the upper limb and trunk: stool seating; printing; table football; pool; darts, woodwork and metal work activities within the heavy workshop.

A standing-frame can prove useful for some of these activities, allowing the paraplegic a period of standing while exercising.

INCOMPLETE LESIONS

Treatment within the occupational therapy department may include activities to encourage strengthening of the lower limbs to increase standing tolerance and to give walking practice. Some examples are: therapeutic bicycle, treadle lathes, fretsaws and working at benches.

People sustaining incomplete paraplegia with minimum residual disability, often of bladder or bowel function, frequently require considerable support and understanding. Although the disability is minimum, to them the 'little missing' is great and the problem apparently insurmountable.

MANAGEMENT OF SENSORY LOSS

It is essential to maintain a good skin condition of those areas where sensation has been altered or lost. Paraplegics — like most people — need only to be made aware of possible danger and the basic 'dos' and 'don'ts' to see the whole purpose and sense of the exercise, but there are also exceptions to this rule.

Examples are as follows.

Clothing

Tight-fitting garments and close-fitting styles, particularly around the waist and in the groin, should be avoided.

The buttons on the back pockets on trousers should be removed.

Shoes should be loose-fitting and easy to put on.

If perspiration is a problem, then clothing should be made of natural rather than synthetic material.

Activity

Table heights should be checked for adequate knee clearance and such items as clamps, when used, should be inverted.

Shoes should always be worn, as these protect the feet from knocks and bumps.

In kitchen work care with hot ovens, hot dishes and hot pipes should all be illustrated.

Before transferring, areas should be checked for foreign bodies — for example, a screwdriver or cigarette lighter.

Fires

Patients must be warned of the dangers incurred by sitting too close to an open, electric or gas fire, radiator or car heater. Care must be taken with the unguarded use of hot-water bottles in cold weather.

Inspection

A paraplegic patient should be taught to inspect regularly his, or her, own skin for signs of pressure or abrasion. If the patient cannot manage this, then relatives must be asked to do so. Use of a mirror and inspection of underpants or bottom bed-sheet for strange marks are two of the easiest and most obvious methods.

Some paraplegic patients find it difficult to understand or accept that the part of the body which they cannot feel must be cared for and must not be ignored.

HOME RESETTLEMENT

At units, such as the Spinal Unit at the Robert Jones and Agnes Hunt Hospital in Oswestry, where there is an established resettlement service, a day visit home with the patients can be arranged together with relatives, and representatives invited to attend from local services such as social services, community nursing or housing, as well as the general practitioner. At Oswestry this visit takes place approximately 4 weeks after mobilisation, or when the patient is able safely to undertake a car journey, and has some understanding and insight into his or her disability and its implications.

Decisions are made on the following:

(a) The suitability of the house for the wheelchair person with minimum, if any, alteration.

(b) Whether the existing house would be suitable with major alterations or extensions — for example, interfloor or stair lift or major reconstruction work.

(c) Whether rehousing is required. Care and attention must be paid not only to the need for independent functioning, but also to the support and friendship offered by neighbours and nearby family and friends, before the complete uprooting of the patient and family is finally decided upon.

(d) Whether, if necessary, it would be possible for a paraplegic patient safely to live alone.

Typical home problems include:

Access with steps or steep incline.

Narrow doorways or restricted turning spaces into rooms within the house.

WC/bathroom upstairs or inaccessible.

Bed and mattress too low and soft, which makes independent dressing, transfers and turning difficult.

Differences in surface heights.

Plan

The house is assessed for its suitability for reasonable access for a weekend at home. Basic criteria are a bed downstairs with adequate mattress; accessible WC or suitable commode provided, with some degree of privacy; and adequate preparation or teaching of relatives if their assistance is required.

Weekends at home are encouraged, as they allow a gradual and controlled reintroduction to life outside the hospital and independence in often less than ideal circumstances. Relatives and friends are able to become acclimatised to differences in life, attitudes and abilities, and the paraplegics themselves enjoy the change from a 7 to a 5 day week in hospital.

A period of 10 days at home follows and, if satisfactory, the patient is discharged soon afterwards.

Routine check-ups are arranged for 1–3 months later and regularly thereafter.

If for any reason resettlement at home is not possible, then a suitable or acceptable alternative arrangement must be made, preferably within the patient's home area, so that family and friends may have access for visiting.

If weekends at home are desirable but not possible because of nursing requirements, inaccessible facilities or a relative's suspected inability to cope, then an occupational therapy assessment flat provides supervised independence and privacy but with help at hand if required.

TRANSPORT

Most paraplegics are perfectly capable of driving a suitably adapted car and should be given encouragement and advice on the best way to set about doing this. Advice is given on:

(a) The financial aspect of purchasing a new or second-hand car and the many schemes that are available to help with this if necessary, often involving use of the Mobility Allowance (see Chapter 9).

(b) The type of car which is needed. An automatic car is recommended and is much easier to drive. Although manual gear-change cars can be converted, the cost is very high and the economics of running the car will be little different compared with the automatic. Discussion must take place as to the most suitable model for the patient. Potential drivers must be encouraged to think in terms of a reliable, practical car, rather than a showy, large and expensive model. A two-door car is easier for access and for loading a wheelchair into the back-seat space. Boot space adequate for storage of the folded wheelchair must also be considered, together with the possible use of the car by other family members or pets.

(c) The types of hand control that are available, with addresses of suppliers and fitting agents, together with details of cost.

(d) The legal requirements of driving with a disability, such as notification of the disability to the Vehicle Licensing Authority, with subsequent amendment made to the driving licence; and notification to the insurance company providing cover for the car.

(e) The various allowances available and vehicle licence redemption schemes operating.

(f) Information on obtaining driving lessons. Many of the larger cities have schools of motoring with ready-adapted automatic cars for disabled learner drivers. Most other driving instructors are only too pleased to teach disabled drivers — but the learner must use his adapted car for driving lessons.

(g) Consideration of local servicing facilities and availability of spare parts, especially if buying a foreign car.

Initial discussion about cars usually takes place informally and spontaneously, when basic facts and requirements are presented for consideration and absorption on the part of the paraplegic and relatives. This first introduction is closely followed by a second, with more detailed information, leaflets, addresses and practical advice and assistance. Patients living locally are only too pleased to demonstrate their own cars and to provide test-driving facilities.

A useful 'litmus' test to measure a paraplegic's acceptance of disability and its actual implications is to talk about driving and the need to modify cars with the use of hand controls. An indifferent response to the subject of 'driving' usually indicates a person who has not yet accepted the fact of 'different' driving and disability.

WORK RESETTLEMENT

There is a close liaison between occupational therapy departments and the Disablement Resettlement Officer (DRO) regarding the suitability of all paraplegics for re-employment. Occupational therapists provide information on a patient's acceptance of disability; particular interests; abilities or skills. They provide facilities for assessment of employment potential, such as concentration, ability to accept direction and to follow instructions, safe handling of tools, timekeeping, enthusiasm and learning abilities.

The DRO liaises with his counterpart in the patient's home area to arrange some suitable form of re-employment or retraining when the patient is discharged.

Re-employment and being able to get to a job is often a useful persuading factor in encouraging a paraplegic to drive again.

SOCIAL CONFIDENCE

The development of social skills and confidence in paraplegics is becoming increasingly important in treatment considerations. The speed and efficiency of the Early Unit treatment often means that independence is gained so quickly that a paraplegic's acceptance of the disability (and its implications) and other people's reaction to it is left far behind the physical rate of progress. Without care and support, these patients can be discharged home inadequately prepared for the challenge of life outside the relative security of a hospital routine.

Within a hospital, a paraplegic's day is planned, with directions to be followed from the moment of wakening. Occupational therapy has the facilities not only to implement recognised methods of treatment, but also to provide a welcoming, natural, friendly and relaxed atmosphere, with every opportunity for the patient to 'unwind' and act 'normally'. Patients and paraplegics, in particular, appreciate this, and their regular unplanned, as well as planned, visits to the department confirm this.

Departmental facilities must be made available to any mobile paraplegics during normal working hours. In this way they become known to all grades of staff, including helpers, students and technicians. No patient should be 'forced' to do anything immediately – if patients do not feel threatened, they relax. A conducted explanatory tour of all facilities, including the inevitable cup of tea, will help to make them feel welcomed. They then return with ideas for activities, questions needing answers, and enthusiasm. Family and friends unexpectedly visiting should be welcomed into the department to observe treatment; but where local visiting becomes regular, then a gentle request can be made to come late in the afternoon.

In this informal atmosphere paraplegics learn to mix with patients with a variety of disabilities from other wards and there can be much useful exchange of ideas and information, either in informal conversation or in more formally organised yet still 'informal' chats. Patients find the atmosphere encouraging and conducive to discussion on personal topics or worries, and know that, if they approach the therapist, time will be made for listening and advice given.

LEISURE PURSUITS

With the problems of unemployment ever increasing, re-employment for a paraplegic is sometimes difficult, if not impossible. Part of a therapist's role is to introduce a patient to ideas for facilitating and developing leisure pursuits, hobbies, sport, etc., which can be followed up and carried out at home after discharge. The last part of every afternoon can be given over to craft, hobbies and sport sessions, when, regardless of other considerations, paraplegic patients can 'have a go' at any activity they wish — art, cookery, gardening, photography, dressmaking, wood turning and crafts, to mention but a few. Every day a different sport can be organised and participation encouraged. Sport has considerable treatment value — balance, strength, co-ordination, concentration, individual striving or team spirit — but sport can also provide a good interest to be followed up with a local club at home, as well as membership of the unit sports club.

Without the companionship of fellow patients and staff, together with their support and encouragement, and without the organisation and discipline of a hospital day, a paraplegic patient can flounder at home, become depressed, bored and despondent, with all the related changes that consequently follow.

Provision of a range of activities and the confidence to 'have a go' at something helps greatly to overcome this type of depression.

INFORMATION SERVICES

The value of working on a small unit ensures that patients get to know each other and gain considerable confidence in the staff. At Oswestry an 'open door' system operates within the occupational therapy department for the provision of information about anything related to disability — cars, holidays, equipment, aids, adaptations, etc. Patients themselves also provide much useful information.

CONCLUSION

Progress in rehabilitation with paraplegic patients is mainly one of a greatly reduced period of hospital care, and much quicker and more intensive rehabilitation and resettlement. With the speed-up of transfer, however, there may be a danger that there is less time to widen patients' interests and to provide more skills and adaptability – for example, the importance of teaching patients to transfer from more than one direction so that they are confident to work out an alternative safe method. Concentrated effort by the therapist to achieve rehabilitation and prevent pressure sores must not extinguish the patient's ability to experiment and adapt.

Occupational therapy can and should provide a valuable contribution to the satisfactory and fulfilling rehabilitation of a paraplegic patient, both from within the treatment and care team and from the individual therapist during hospital care and after discharge.

For practical information see Appendixes. See also Chapter 9 on types of housing and transport.

6. The role of the medical social worker

Gelia Kirkby

The National Spinal Injuries Centre was opened in 1944 and is part of the Stoke Mandeville General Hospital. In the summer of 1983, the Spinal Centre moved to a purpose-built building, still based within the hospital grounds. The money to build the new centre was raised by public donations. The design and layout of the Spinal Centre reflects a progressive and flexible policy towards the present and future needs of spinal patients in terms of physical care, rehabilitation and research. There is an increasing emphasis on social rehabilitation which is exemplified in the creation of a communal dining area, private family rooms, and a leisure and educational room furnished with educational video equipment.

Of the patients admitted to the Spinal Centre approximately one-third are paraplegic and the remainder are tetraplegic (sometimes known as *quadriplegic*).

The social worker is part of the rehabilitation team, which includes doctors, nurses, physiotherapists and occupational therapists. However, owing to staff shortages, the occupational therapists only treat the tetraplegics, the most severely disabled.

The social work involvement with paraplegic and tetraplegic patients is limited because of the large volume of work assigned to a small team of social workers. My perception, therefore, of the social work role is a fusion between a service that would be given if more social workers were available and the frustrating reality.

In essence the social work task covers four main areas:

(1) To offer social work support and counselling to patients and their families through the use of individual and family interviews.

(2) To provide the rehabilitation team with an assessment of family functioning, home environment and community facilities.

(3) To provide practical information on matters such as housing adaptations, DHSS benefits and local resources for the physically handicapped.

(4) To liaise between the hospital rehabilitation team and the community care team.

These four areas are not mutually exclusive, and one way of describing the social work role is intermittently to illustrate it with the case history of Alex.

At the age of 31 Alex was involved in a road traffic accident and as a result became a paraplegic. He and his wife Jenny have two children — Alison, aged 4, and Paul, aged 6. He had worked for 3 years as a sales representative with a computer firm and had recently moved to a three-bedroomed detached house. Alex was admitted to his local general hospital and 3 days later transferred to the Spinal Unit at Stoke Mandeville Hospital.

HOSPITAL TRANSFERS

Transfer from one hospital to another adds to the frequently felt shock and confusion of the patient, because there is additional adjustment to a new hospital environment, staff nursing routine and patient community. Often the family have a 100 mile journey and the distance increases the patient's sense of estrangement and homesickness.

A further complicating factor involving hospital transfer is that the staff are often unsure as to what information has been given to the patient and the family before the transfer, and whether this has facilitated or inhibited their perception of the Spinal Unit as being rehabilitative rather than providing a 'cure' for spinal injuries. The family will have to adjust to sharing for many months the caring role of the Unit, and this may arouse anxiety and suspicion if previous hospital experiences have led them to see the medical staff as authoritarian, clinical and uncaring.

COMMUNICATION

All newly injured people are automatically seen by the social worker, and the preferred first contact is to be present when the consultant tells the patient and his family of the diagnosis. This means that all concerned understand the medical condition, and this joint meeting conveys two messages, one explicit and the other implicit.

The first message is an explicit demonstration of open communication between team members, patient and family, and serves as a model for future contact. The second message is implicit in that the presence of a social worker, whose prime concern is the well-being of the patient, with the doctor, whose first responsibility is the patient's physical condition, is acknowledging the patient as an integrated whole.

With all the team knowing the degree of injury, the family is freed to start the long process of adjustment.

FAMILY ATTITUDES

It is important that the social worker gains an understanding of the patient and his family. This is assisted by taking a comprehensive social history which details the family's and patient's developmental history. The social worker needs to know the pre-injury attitude towards and experience of disability. Unfortunately, the commonly held view is a negative one, disability being synonymous with low intellect, poor job prospects, inadequate housing and general unhappiness.

Apart from factual information, the social worker needs to be aware of the pre-existing family and patient stress and loss, such as marital conflict and separation, alcoholism, redundancy, death, severe financial problems, anxieties about children, and previous mental and physical ill-health in key members of the immediate or extended family. Previous crisis, the impact and how it was handled, will give a good indication as to the likely reaction to disability.

Crises are likely to occur at transition points, and usually involve a change of role, such as becoming a parent or becoming unemployed. For many people, transition points are negotiated with minimal support from family and friends. However, in a crisis which is caused by sudden transfer from a state of active physical well-being to partial paralysis, social work involvement is necessary if only to provide practical assistance.

Caplan (1961) identifies a crisis as being a short-term upset in emotional equilibrium, resulting in anxiety, tension and cognitive confusion. Thus, temporarily, the ability to cope and adjust to their new situation is beyond the patient's and the family's capacity.

One way of helping the family to mobilise their emotional and intellectual abilities is by the rehabilitation team giving basic information about physical, psychological and social aspects of disability. Alternatively, the presence and the accessibility of the staff and the social worker provides reassurance and demonstrates acceptance of the patient and his family during the early stage of acute distress and unhappiness.

HOSPITALISATION

From 4 to 6 months in hospital for a paraplegic patient might present a threat to family unity, but this will depend upon the nature of the pre-injury family relationships of caring and cohesion. The change in economic stability, and disruption of familial roles and habits, will vary according to the status of the patient.

In the case of Alex his economic and parental responsibilities were partially suspended, and while immobilised in bed, he was the dependent, passive recipient of nursing and medical care, while Jenny assumed the role of independent organiser.

Independence versus dependence, and autonomy versus integration, are central issues in all interpersonal relationships. However, these personal issues become clouded by cultural attitudes which give high regard to and make independence and its close companion, control, virtuous. Independence, dependence, autonomy and integration are not static states but vary with each social encounter and personal relationship.

In common with other patients, Alex was confined to bed and flat on his back for 10 weeks, which meant that, apart from loss of sensation in the lower limbs, impaired bladder, bowel and genital functioning, he had further deprivation due to restricted environmental and social stimulus.

When lying flat, the patient's field of vision is limited and the ability to communicate is severely hampered. However, when the patient is immobile, it enables the staff and the social worker to form a bond and encourage self-motivation and a sense of purpose about the future. The social worker can help the patient both in terms of the initial experience of disability and to make sense of the hospital environment, using it as a positive experience despite a sense of powerlessness which institutional procedures and policies tend to evoke.

COUNSELLING

Although counselling is, rightly, not the sole prerogative of the social worker, to offer effective counselling it is important to avoid the trap of overidentification and to examine self-attitude towards serious disability and loss. As with any significant loss, a person needs time to mourn its passing. Mourning is a healing reaction which allows an individual to give up the past, enjoy the present achievements and pursue the future. Although the concepts of mourning vary in detail, the phases, in general, are shock and denial, aggression and despair, acceptance and resolution. The last stage is concerned with adjustment, and while I accept criticism of the able-bodied professionals who feel that all disabled people should be depressed (clinically), there is an emotional journey before resolution and adjustment are made, be it to paralysis, redundancy or divorce. Adjustment will be facilitated by the patient's having a stable family, a sound education or salable work skills, financial security, determination, flexibility and humour. In brief, those patients who were coping reasonably well with life prior to injury have a greater probability of adjusting to spinal injury.

PHYSICAL REHABILITATION

Once the patient is mobile in a wheelchair, active physical rehabilitation begins. Rehabilitation is the long process of enabling a disabled person to resume a normal life — physically, socially and psychologically. It starts on admission, and the social and psychological rehabilitation continues long after discharge.

The central focus of the rehabilitation team is the patient, and ideally he and his family should be involved in setting goals for rehabilitation. Specialist roles can lead to the patient's being given possibly conflicting goals. Mutually agreed goals are therefore important; otherwise, conflicting expectations can reduce the effectiveness of the rehabilitation programme. The team needs to understand and value each other's contribution and, while acknowledging each specialist area, must not feel professionally threatened when these areas overlap.

The staff expect the patient to be motivated, 'motivation' being a term often used by the rehabilitation team to denote co-operation, on the assumption that, if the patient is motivated, he will co-operate. However, some individuals choose not to attend certain therapy sessions because the activity holds no meaning and cannot be related to personal goals such as returning to work or running the home. An activity which is perceived as meaningless will not be sustained, and it is the joint responsibility of the team and the patient to reassess the rehabilitation goals.

Within the rehabilitation team the social worker occupies a privileged position in bridging the gap between the hospital and the community, and so is able to present and explain the contribution of each to the other.

There is a need for the rehabilitation and community teams to recognise the totality of the situation, and the social worker is able to collate information concerning family functioning and community resources. In common with other assessments such as physical progress, the social work assessment is fluid because the patient and the family are adapting as each day highlights another dimension of the disability, but an assessment needs to be made in order to decide what community agencies, if any, the patient should be referred to.

WEEKEND LEAVE

Once medically fit, a patient is encouraged to spend a weekend at home because weekend leave is seen as a necessary and integral part of the rehabilitation programme (see Chapter 5). It helps to reduce institutionalisation and dependency, and allows the family and friends to acclimatise to the disability. Weekend leave also shows whether skills learnt in the Unit, whether in physical care or mobility, need to be adapted to the individual patient's life style and home.

Alex found on his weekend leaves that within the secure and familiar environment of his home and community he began to redefine his role, personally as a husband, father and son, and socially as a neighbour, racing-car enthusiast and ratepayer. This was a painful time, and Alex and his family were aware that society viewed him as being different from and less able than his former self, a message which was conveyed by attitudes and physical inaccessibility to old haunts. However, at a personal level, re-establishing contacts with friends, neighbours and work colleagues was a gratifying experience. Negotiating passages, doorways and furniture came with practice, and to create extra space the children were reminded not to leave toys strewn across the floor. The dog was trained, rather unsuccessfully, not to lie at her master's feet in front of the wheelchair.

ADAPTATIONS

The Spinal Unit social worker is responsible for contacting the community occupational therapist who assesses the house for adaptations (see Chapters 4, 5, 9). Under the Chronically Sick and Disabled Persons Act 1970 the local authority social services department have a duty to provide aids and, where appropriate, finance adaptations which are necessary for a disabled person. For council house tenants the housing department is responsible for the cost of the structural adaptations, and under the Housing Act 1970 provision is made for owner occupiers to receive from a local authority improvement and intermediate grants. Rate relief is also granted on any addition or feature to the house for the disabled person, such as an additional bathroom, lavatory or bedroom, or central heating.

Alex's house required ramps, the widening of several doorways, the fitting of a hand-rail in the bathroom to aid transfers and the installation of a stair-lift. Until these modifications had been carried out, he made use of a commode and slept in the dining-room. Having to 'make do', with its attendant loss of privacy, is an all too common aspect of disability, especially for the newly disabled.

Unfortunately, when the environment is not adapted to physical needs, the disability becomes a handicap which expands or contracts according to the architectural conditions.

SEX COUNSELLING

Like many couples with young children, Alex and Jenny occupied traditional roles, in that he was involved in the competitive stressful world of work, while she created a warm environment and coped with the daily demands of two children.

The artificial divide between the sexes, caricatured as rational, unemotional, assertive male and intuitive, emotional, passive female is made irrelevant by the trauma of a spine-injured man who, during the process of adjustment, becomes more conscious of his emotions.

Whether the individual feels detached, overwhelmed, depressed or psychologically more complete depends upon the capacity for emotional growth and willingness to take emotional risks through self-disclosure. For some, being disabled becomes a way of life which dominates all thoughts and actions, whereas for others it becomes a viable reason for

obstructive feelings of anger or helplessness. However, disability can also cause some patients to channel an aimless or
cavalier attitude towards life into an involved and purposeful
approach.

Alex's feelings of dependence and doubts about self-worth
were further compounded by the sexual aspects of paralysis,
which question the stereotype virile, athletic male.

Sexual performance is a sensitive area, and in order to
explore its dimensions the patient and his partner need to
have a secure, honest and easy relationship with someone
who feels comfortable with his or her own sexuality. It is
essential that the counsellor have factual knowledge about
the physical implications of the paralysis. Also, the counsellor
needs to understand what sex means to the patient and what
it represents to the relationship, and to place its expression
within the total caring relationship as shown through warmth,
concern, companionship and respect (see Chapter 7).

CARE GROUPS

The hospital social worker, in conjunction with other members of the team, helps to run a series of groups for those
patients who wish to discuss informally with the staff and
other patients topics such as skin care, mobility, pressure
groups for the disabled, work, DHSS benefits, family relationships and children. Sometimes ex-patients are invited to the
group, the aim being to share their experience of being
disabled and offer practical advice.

Study days can be organised for relatives of newly injured
patients hosted by the hospital social worker. Other members
of staff are invited to give talks on subjects such as body care,
spasms and house adaptations which supplement the information previously given by the rehabilitation team. Study
days enable relatives to meet one another; to share anxieties;
to meet ex-patients to hear how they organise their lives, and
whether they work, have a family or have married since the
injury. The relatives of newly injured patients find it helpful
to meet ex-patients and to realise that disability does not
dominate their lives.

DISABLEMENT RESETTLEMENT OFFICER
INVOLVEMENT

Once weekend visits have been established, the patient can often approach and appraise work in a constructive manner. It is at this stage that the Disablement Resettlement Officer (DRO) should be approached and the social worker is the main source of referral (see Chapter 8). The timing of the referral is important, because patients preoccupied with bladders or demoralised because toilet transfers have yet to be achieved are not mentally receptive to the world of work. The main task of the DRO is to help the patient identify problems regarding work, to liaise with the employer and, where appropriate, organise retraining.

For many disabled people one of the key components for their former occupation was ease of mobility, as required by nurses, car mechanics, electricians, labourers or milkmen. However, depending upon personality, intellect and previous work skills, retraining can be total or sufficient to enable a person to extend an area of knowledge and thereby obtain work.

Alex was fortunate in that his employer was willing to re-arrange his work routine because he was reliable, competent and well liked, but, more importantly, working in 'computers' meant that he had a job that required mental rather than physical skill.

The computer industry is ideally suited to disabled people, and the British Computer Society has founded a specialist group for the disabled with the aim of training and employing handicapped people, some of whom can work from home with a direct telephone link to a computer.

For Alex, one of the hardest parts of returning to work was accepting help from other colleagues in order to overcome architectural barriers, such as stairs which could not be ramped. He was also concerned that having less mobility might be viewed as a factor against promotion and that certain career opportunities would now be closed. Work had been central to his life and identity, and Alex had always measured success in terms of salary and career advancement. Just before discharge he was beginning to re-evaluate these beliefs.

RETURN TO THE COMMUNITY

However keen a person is to return home, discharge means going from partial dependence on skilled professional help and companionship of other disabled people to managing on one's own and often being the only disabled person in the immediate neighbourhood. It would be beneficial if, prior to discharge, the Unit social worker, with another member of the team, arranged a meeting in the patient's home with the community care team, the patient and the family, in order to exchange information and make any necessary plans. However, the geographical distance, and shortage of staff, usually results in liaison being conducted on the telephone, but the patient can, and does, meet the rehabilitation team, either formally at a case conference or informally as individuals, to discuss physical progress and future care. Social and emotional rehabilitation is only in the early stages on discharge.

Alex, having learned physical independence, on his final return home had then to acquire tolerance and flexibility to cope with an environment not aware of the disabled. In order to re-establish himself as the family breadwinner and useful member of the community, he had to challenge the social handicaps of disability — this he had begun to do when seen by the social worker at his out-patient appointment.

VOLUNTARY ORGANISATIONS

Unfortunately, unless the patient lives within the hospital catchment area, time and distance prevent any member of the rehabilitation team from following the patient into the community. The Spinal Unit team are aware, however, that short-term continuity of care could help reduce some physical, social and emotional problems. It is unfortunate that these problems currently often go unaided, as the majority of families do not refer themselves to the Social Services Department but prefer to resolve difficulties with the help of family, friends or their doctor. Thus, apart from the initial involvement of the community occupational therapist, district nurse or general practitioner, professional carers are not often involved in the lives of paraplegic patients.

Nevertheless, depending upon need, a person can join a local social club for the disabled or become a member of one of the voluntary societies, such as the Spinal Injuries Association, the Disability Alliance or The Royal Association for Disability and Rehabilitation, which give information and advice. The degree of involvement, if any, with an organisation specialising in the welfare of disabled people will partly reflect the wish to bring about change in attitude and facilities, the need for companionship, support and the awareness of what the impact of disability means to the disabled individual. Some useful contacts are given in the Appendixes.

CONCLUSION

In this chapter the scope of social work intervention may have appeared to ignore the inherent difficulties for any social worker working in a hospital where frequently social work skills and contributions are difficult to evaluate against the concrete reality of giving a bed-bath, examining a patient or teaching a transfer. Time scales and values differ in that social workers tend to adopt a long-term perspective and do not expect problems, the majority of which have a long history, to be solved quickly, whereas the medical profession requires that the problem be solved sufficiently to allow discharge. Both attitudes are valid and raise the complicated issue of what constitutes health care.

Within the context of the rehabilitation team, the social worker can assist the patient to make full use of the facilities offered and help to make the experience of being in hospital a positive one, which will influence subsequent contact with the medical profession. The essential role of the social worker is to mediate between the patient and the community, and to help lay the foundations for adjustment to disability without rancour.

For practical information see Appendixes.

REFERENCE

Caplan, G. (1961). *An Approach to Community Mental Health*, Tavistock, London.

BIBLIOGRAPHY

Eisenberg, H. G. and Falconer, J. A. (1978). *Treatment of the Spinal Cord Injury — An Interdisciplinary Perspective*, Charles C. Thomas, Springfield, Ill.
Fallon, B. (1975). *So You're Paralysed. . .* , Spinal Injuries Association, London.
Mooney, T., Cole, T. and Chilgren, R. (1975). *Sexual Options for Paraplegics and Quadriplegics*, Little Brown, Boston.
Rabin, B. (1980). *The Sensuous Wheeler*, Joyce, Multi Media Resource Centre, San Francisco.
Trieschmann, R. B. (1980). *Spinal Cord Injuries — Psychological, Social and Vocational Adjustment*, Pergamon Press, Oxford and New York.

7. The role of modern sex therapy applied to paraplegia

Graham Powell

INTRODUCTION

In this chapter sex therapy is considered in physical and psychological terms. The sex act comprises several distinct stages, each of which can be considered later in relation to paraplegia.

(1) *Sex drive, libido or sexual arousability.* This is the appetitive motivation from which sexual activity springs. The drive varies from individual to individual, depending upon factors such as hormonal levels, attitudes acquired during upbringing, the nature and success of previous sexual experiences, and short-term parameters such as opportunity, anxiety and stress. There is some evidence that libido is higher in man than in woman. The preferred frequency of intercourse, for example, is 4.8 times per week for husbands but only 3.8 for wives (Fisher, 1973), although the actual frequency might be somewhat lower, at 2-3 times a week (e.g. Kinsey *et al.*, 1953), since libidinal feelings do not always coincide.

(2) *Elicitation of arousal.* The stimuli precipitating arousal may be external, involving direct touching of sensitive aspects of the genitalia, or internal or psychogenic, meaning erotic thoughts and fantasies. Arousal is evidenced in men by vasocongestion and erection, and in women by vasocongestion and vaginal lubrication controlled by parasympathetic roots from between S2 and S3. Other psychogenic factors, especially anxiety, can substantially reduce, or inhibit entirely, the arousal response.

(3) *Ejaculation in men*. This is the emission of semen from the erect penis in, perhaps, five or ten pulses. Semen can also exude before this phase and also from the limp penis, a full erection not being a vital prerequisite. Once the ejaculation has begun, it proceeds irrevocably and is not under voluntary control or under influence of psychogenic factors.

(4) *Orgasms*. Cognitively this appears to be the same for both men and women, involving ecstatic feelings, loss of body boundary, a lowering of pain thresholds, and various other strong emotions. Orgasm in men usually coincides with ejaculation, after which there is a loss of erection and a refractory phase in which the penis fails to respond to normally arousing stimuli. In women orgasm is accompanied by involuntary contractions of the vaginal and pelvic muscles, which does not lead to a refractory phase (Masters and Johnson, 1966). Ejaculation and orgasm are controlled by sympathetic supplies from between L1 and L2.

Finally, since we are concerned with a specific disability, paraplegia, we must also consider a fifth aspect of the sex act, viz. coitus.

(5) *Fertility*. In men this depends mainly on the number of viable spermatozoa found in the semen, and in women upon proper ovulation and viable ova production. This may not be an aspect uppermost in the minds of individuals engaged in coitus, but it is an important background factor, being a psychogenic variable inhibiting sex drive in some couples. For example, it has been noted in sterilisation clinics that the operation can have an immediate negative impact on both partners' interest in sex, with patients complaining they no longer feel totally masculine or totally feminine.

These five elements constitute a *loosely* coupled system, for the absence of any one item does not completely predict the absence of any other item, and, similarly, the presence of any item does not completely ensure the presence of any other item. Therefore, for example, there can be ejaculation without orgasm, erection without arousal, prolonged arousal without orgasm, and so on.

From this it tends to follow that the effects of paraplegia can be various, and we are only just beginning to understand which aspects of the sex act are disrupted by which spinal lesions. A review of the literature suggests that paraplegia influences sexual functioning in the following ways, taking each of the above five points in turn.

(1) *Paraplegia and libido.* It cannot be supposed that most spinal lesions directly affect those hormones and endocrines that facilitate sexual preparedness. In any case, sexual feelings and behaviour in humans (or animal analogues) can continue in the absence of normal sex hormones such as androgen, especially if the person (or animal analogue) is sexually experienced, with an established pattern of sexual behaviour (see Paintin, 1976, for a brief but clear review of the physiology of sex). Therefore, loss of libido in paraplegia is much more likely to be due to secondary cognitive factors such as loss of sexual confidence. Paraplegics are not, then, sexually 'inert'; they are liable to have normal sexual urges needing fulfilment.

(2) *Paraplegia and arousal signs.* Most research here has concentrated upon the male, because arousal is relatively easily measured by observing the erectile responses of the penis. In contrast, female arousal is more difficult to assess: by thermal conduction in vaginal tissues, say, or vaginal reflectance as detected by a photocell (Gillan and Brindley, 1979).

There are, as mentioned previously, two kinds of erection to consider — reflexive and psychogenic. According to Brindley (1982), reflex erections to direct stimulation of the glans and shaft of the penis are to be expected in most cases unless sacral segments of the cord are destroyed.

Psychogenic erections are much less common, reported in 4 out of 77 cases of complete cervical lesions (Bors and Comars, 1960) and 42 out of 251 cases with complete lesions below T8 (Comars 1970). The reports of the 4 cervical cases are doubted by Brindley (1982), who points out that psychogenic erections need to be mediated by roots between T9 and L4. Instead, Brindley puts the observations of Bors and Comars down to inaccurate observation coupled with unnoticed and accidental direct stimulation.

In sum, the male paraplegic in his sexual activity has by and large to make use of reflex erections. This is a most important point, because it explains the root of the paraplegic's performance fear. The normal male can feel sexually confident because an erection is almost invariably obtained *before* direct sexual activity begins. But the paraplegic has to begin sexual activity often *without* an erection and wait for it to develop with contact. The natural fear is that the erection will not arrive. The impact of this kind of worry cannot be underestimated, because in normals it can readily lead to impotence (Masters and Johnson, 1970).

(3) *Paraplegia and ejaculation.* There are three means of eliciting ejaculation to consider. Through ordinary sexual means (i.e. manual, oral or vaginal stimulation) about 8 per cent of paraplegics can reach ejaculation (Zeitlin *et al.*, 1957; Bors and Comars, 1960; Comars, 1970). The best rate (about 10 per cent) is with lower thoracic and lumbar cases, and the lowest rate (about 4 per cent) is with cervical cases. The second means involves the extra-strong stimulation provided by a vibrator. Brindley (1982) combines the data of Francois *et al.* (1980) and Brindley (1981a) to obtain a success rate of around 70 per cent. Third, we have electroejaculation (Horne *et al.*, 1948; Brindley, 1981b). This technique consists of stimulating the lateral wall of the penis (via the rectum) at either the right or left obturator point. Unlike the vibrator method, in which an erection is always produced, an erection is not always seen. The emission of semen is also different, being at best a trickling discharge.

Of Brindley's 92 cases, 42 exhibited external semen (exuded from the penis) and 14 showed only retrograde semen (discharged into the bladder and found later in the patient's urine). Electroejaculation, because it can cause severe pain (depending on the completeness and position of the lesion), is sometimes undertaken under general anaesthetic.

(4) *Paraplegia and orgasm.* Comars (1970) found that 21 of his 251 male cases reported orgasms, but their quality and intensity is unknown.

(5) *Paraplegia and fertility.* The depressingly low fertility of paraplegic men has been pinpointed as a major source of marital dissatisfaction (David *et al.*, 1977). However, improved methods of semen collection can increase the probability of

pregnancy (Brindley, 1981a, b; 1982). For example, within the 14 couples who used Brindley's vibratory ejaculation or electroejaculation at home, 4 wives are pregnant to date. Further, there is some suggestion from Brindley (1982) that fertility as judged by the number of mobile spermatozoa per ejaculate *increases* with successive electrojaculates.

The dual aim of sex therapy is to increase a couple's enjoyment of sex and to reduce the couple's dysfunction. Implicit in this definition is the notion that the *couple* should be counselled whenever possible, not just the one person who feels responsible (i.e. not just the *paraplegic*). To make this clear, consider the attitude of a paraplegic's wife quoted by David *et al.* (1977):

Q. 'Do you enjoy sexual intercourse with your husband?'
A. 'Can you imagine all the possible secretions, smells and other things that one has to suffer in order to get a very small amount of sexual gratification?'

Here is a woman obviously repulsed by many aspects of available sexual behaviours with very low aspirations for their enjoyability. Sex taking place in this atmosphere is almost certainly doomed to failure. Therefore, to some extent this wife's attitude would be labelled 'the dysfunction' as much as the husband's paraplegia. There are also interactional factors of course — what did this husband do to reduce the likelihood of 'secretions, smells and other things'?

Modern sex therapy depends first upon an accurate and multi-baselined assessment of sexual functioning. Questions are asked, and measures taken, of *behaviour* (things the couple do or do not do, habits and routines), *cognitions* (attitudes, knowledge, beliefs, fantasies, hopes, fears and emotions) and *physiological responses* (sources and types of stimulation, physical reactions, anxiety symptoms, arousal and signs). Within each of these categories there are behaviours that need *reinforcing* and others that need *eliminating*; cognitions that need *fostering* and others that need *undermining*; physiological responses that require *enhancing* and others that need *diminishing*. This gives us a six-fold framework (see table 7.1) for (a) analysis of the problem, (b)

Table 7.1 Outline of a systematic approach to sexual counselling

	Aspects to accelerate		Aspects to decelerate	
Behaviours	Problem areas	$= x, y, x, \ldots$	Problem areas	$= x, y, z, \ldots$
	Treatment targets	$= X, Y, Z$	Treatment targets	$= X, Y, Z$
	Treatment methods	$= ??$	Treatment methods	$= ??$
Cognitions	Problem areas	$= x, y, z, \ldots$	Problem areas	$= x, y, z, \ldots$
	Treatment targets	$= X, Y, Z$	Treatment targets	$= X, Y, Z$
	Treatment methods	$= ??$	Treatment methods	$= ??$
Physiology	Problem areas	$= x, y, z, \ldots$	Problem areas	$= x, y, z, \ldots$
	Treatment targets	$= X, Y, Z$	Treatment targets	$= X, Y, Z$
	Treatment methods	$= ??$	Treatment methods	$= ??$

establishment of treatment targets and (c) selection of treatment methods. These three superordinate stages can now be briefly described, each with special reference to paraplegia.

ANALYSIS OF THE PROBLEM

No single interview schedule can ever be fully comprehensive and fit all requirements, but here are some of the most relevant questions to ask and measures to take. It should go without saying that those enquiries have to be made of *both* partners:

(a) Behavioural aspects
 History of sexual behaviour
 masturbation
 light petting
 heavy petting
 intercourse
 homosexual contact
 Current sexual activity, including frequency counts
 masturbation
 petting
 intercourse
 homosexual contact
 extra-relationship affairs
 Sex-related activities
 erotic films, books, plays
 discussions on sex
 History of any sexual problems prior to or consequent upon onset of paraplegia, in either patient or patient's partner
 premature ejaculation (men)
 primary impotence (men)
 secondary impotence (men)
 ejaculatory failure (men)
 retarded ejaculation (men)
 loss of libido (men and women)
 poor orgasm (men and women)
 vaginismus (women)

dyspareunia (mainly women)
primary orgasmic dysfunction (women)
sexual deviations (men and women)
General history of current relationship — quality of relationship or marriage
    problems in the relationship
    future of the relationship
General description of social life
    amount of contact with others
    close friends
    adequacy of social skills
    regular social activities enjoyed
Behavioural limitations imposed by paraplegia
(b) Cognitive aspects
    Sex knowledge
        in general (a standard questionnaire may be helpful)
        in relation to effects of paraplegia
    Attitudes to sex and sexual matters
        'conservative' or 'liberal'
        parental attitudes
        views on specific behaviours — for example, oral sex, manual masturbation, etc.
    Libido
        fantasies and daydreams, frequency and nature
        sexual urges, frequency
    Self-confidence and self-esteem
        general
        sexual
    Perceived role of sex in relationships
    Perceived importance of sex for others, especially the partner
    Fears and worries about sexual performance
        relating to self
        relating to partner
    Relevant emotions due to paraplegia
        anger
        frustration
        helplessness
        depression
        etc., etc.
    Perceived reactions of others to paraplegia

(c) Physiological aspects
  Nature of stimuli found to be erotic
    kissing
    deep (French) kissing
    sundry caresses of earlobes, back, feet, etc.
   genital caresses
    penile glans
    penile shaft
    scrotum
    clitoris
    vagina
    rectum
    breasts and nipples
    etc., etc.
   other sensory stimulation
    smells, perfumes
    music
    atmosphere
    words
   nature of arousal responses
    reflex erections (strength, duration, probability)
    psychogenic erections
    reflex vaginal lubrication and vasocongestion of vulva
    psychogenic vaginal lubrication and vasocongestion of
     vulva
   nature and quality of orgasmic sensations
    ways of reaching orgasm
    probability of attaining orgasm
   inhibiting physiological states
    anxiety
    disgust or revulsion

ESTABLISHING TREATMENT TARGETS

From an interview schedule similar to the above a picture of the main problem areas for the couple can be built up. It is simply not possible to list the variety and frequency of problems that can arise with paraplegia, because research reviews in the area have been far too scant in their questioning (Guttman, 1964; Fink *et al.*, 1969; Fitzpatrick, 1972; Griffith *et al.*, 1973; Teal and Atheston, 1975; Berkman *et al.*, 1978; Abrams, 1981).

For the individual couple or for the individual case if there is no partner, a structured list of problem targets can be formulated as presented in table 7.2, for a 24-year-old paraplegic girl (road traffic accident at age 15) with no boy friend. She had had some sexual contact before age 15, involving kissing and touching of breasts, which she had enjoyed. She had never masturbated and never experienced orgasm. It can be seen immediately that in order to tackle her sexual problem, treatment aims have to be much wider. Her sexual problem she defined as follows:

'I want to have sex and babies and I feel sexy sometimes. Boys, though, they're turned off by me. I think they would be, anyway. And what would I do if they, you know, "touched" me. I wouldn't know what to do — I mean I don't know anything about *ordinary* sex, so what do I do like this. As soon as I talk to boys now, I dry up and get really embarrassed 'cos I think about sex straight away. Friends tell me it's OK to use my mouth and hands on them but I'd *die* of embarrassment if it came to that. I don't think I could do it anyway; you know, get stuff all over me. I'd be sick I bet. It won't come to that, though, will it? I don't mind about not having orgasms myself because lots of women don't, do they, but they can still enjoy it, can't they? I thought about asking my mum where to touch a boy to, you know, turn him on; how to touch him. But we've never talked about sex, so I can't ask her. *She'd* die. I'm just not going near boys because I've got all these hang-ups. No one knows, though. Mum thinks I've forgot about sex.'

Her problems are behavioural (avoidance of low-level heterosexual contact and poor social skills), cognitive (attitudes towards manual and oral sex) and physiological (possible anxiety reactions to sexual contact). Specific targets are listed, though not comprehensively, in table 7.2.

Table 7.2 Treatment targets for the 24-year-old female paraplegic

	Things to encourage	Things to discourage

Behaviour	Going to the pub with girl friends
	Going to the cinema
	Accepting invitations to parties
	Social skills:
	  eye contact
	  asking questions
	  answering questions fully
	Personal appearance:
	  buy own clothes (not Mum)
	  go to the dentist
		Saying 'No' to all invitations
		Avoidance of crowds of people
		Avoidance of talking about sex
		  with girl friends
		Social skills:
		  giggling
		  sitting behind everyone

Cognitions	Read a couple of explicit, instructive
	  sex manuals
	Read some amiable 'pornography' to
	  get used to the idea of different
	  kinds of sex activity
	Get used to visualising and fantasising
	  about masturbation and oral sex
	Obtain information about fertility in
	  general and her own in particular
	Ask friends to say, truthfully, how they
	  react to her as a paraplegic
		Various exaggerated negative
		  perceptions of herself, e.g.
		  that her facial attractiveness has
		  somehow diminished because of
		  the paraplegia

Physiology	Exploration by self-touching of any genital
	  response to direct stimulation
		Feelings of intense anxiety and dis-
		  comfort when the thought of sex
		  arises

TREATMENT

Sex counselling and sex therapy tend to shade into each other as far as paraplegia is concerned. Sensible and useful counselling or advice can be given just by analysing the situation properly, but specific therapy skills and techniques will obviously be useful on occasions. The broad texts of Masters and Johnson (1970) and Kaplan (1974) are useful here.

In the behavioural sphere they show the usefulness of graded change by 'homework' assignments reinforced with explicit verbal instructions. A couple's behaviour can also be changed by using a behaviour-contracting approach, in which each person's behaviour is reinforced by the other's (Azrin *et al.*, 1973), or by improving the verbal feedback between couples (Lobitz and Lo Piccolo, 1972) with communication skills training.

In the cognitive sphere confidence and self-esteem can be expected to change, on the assumption that we judge ourselves by what we see ourselves doing (Bem, 1970). Otherwise, attitudes and beliefs can be altered by subtle logical persuasion that minimises psychological reactance (Brehm, 1966), or by the direct giving of information (see Kiesler *et al.*, 1969). Some of the most important cognitions are the paraplegic's perceptions of how others see him or her. These perceptions can only improve in accuracy if there is sufficient first-hand experience of social interaction, which can perhaps be supplied in a group therapy setting.

Finally, as for the physiological area, distaste and anxiety over certain sexual behaviours can be diminished by desensitisation, either in the imagination or *in vivo* (Laughren and Kass, 1975; Wincze and Caird, 1976). It also might be possible to build up certain arousal responses through biofeedback (Barlow *et al.*, 1975) or masturbation training (Langevin and Martin, 1975), or to increase sexual responsiveness in general with a combination of hormonal and psychological treatment (Carney *et al.*, 1978).

CONCLUSION

The sexual problems of paraplegics are not quite the same as those encountered in ordinary sex therapy. However, some problems do overlap, such as the proliferation of avoidance behaviour, the development of inhibiting attitudes, and the suppression of sexual feeling by anxiety and performance fears. The structured and systematic approach of modern sex therapy has something to offer in terms of analysing the paraplegic client's problem and formulating sensible, specific treatment targets. Sometimes, specific sex therapy techniques (such as sensate focusing to reduce embarrassment or imaginal desensitisation to reduce anxiety) can also be useful.

APPENDIX

Sex therapy is today fairly freely available throughout the UK. Referrals are made to sex clinics through the patient's general practitioner, but most clinics will also take referrals from professional aid organisations. Occasionally self-referrals can be made. A list of major sex clinics is given in the back of *Sex Therapy Today*, by Paul R. Gillan, Open Books, London (1976).

REFERENCES

Abrams, K. S. (1981). The impact on marriages of adult-onset paraplegia. *Paraplegia*, 19, 253-259.

Azrin, N. M., Nanter, B. J. and Jones, R. (1973). Reciprocity counselling: a new rapid learning-based procedure for marital counselling. *Behav. Res. Ther.*, 11, 365-382.

Barlow, D. H., Agras, W. S., Abel, G. G., Blanchard, E. B. and Young, L. D. (1975). Biofeedback and reinforcement to increase heterosexual arousal in homosexuals. *Behav. Res. Ther.*, 13, 45-50.

Bem, D. J. (1970). *Beliefs, Attitudes and Human Affairs*, Brooks and Cole, New York.

Berkman, A., Weissman, R. and Frielich, M. (1978). Sexual adjustment of spinal cord injured veterans living in the community. *Arch. phys. Med. Rehab.*, 59, 29-33.

Bors, E. and Comars, A. E. (1980). Neurological disturbance of sexual function with specific reference to 529 patients with spinal cord injury. *Urol. Surv.*, 10, 191-222.

Brehm, J. W. (1966). *A Theory of Psychological Reactance*, Academic Press, New York.

Brindley, G. S. (1981a). Reflex ejaculation under vibratory stimulation in paraplegic men. *Paraplegia*, **19**, 300-303.

Brindley, G. S. (1981b). Electroejaculation: its techniques, neurological implications and uses. *J. Neurol. Neurosurg. Psychiat.*, **44**, 9-18.

Brindley, G. S. (1982). Sexual functioning and fertility in paraplegic men. In *Clinical Practice in Neurology* (Ed. T. B. Hargreave), Springer-Verlag, Berlin.

Carney, A., Bancroft, J. and Matthews, A. (1978). Combination of hormonal and psychological treatment for female sexual unresponsiveness. A comparative study. *Br. J. Psychiat.*, **132**, 339-346.

Comars, A. E. (1970). Sexual function among patients with spinal injury. *Urol. int.*, **23**, 134-168.

David, A., Gur, S. and Razin, R. (1977). Survival in marriage in the paraplegic couple: psychological study. *Paraplegia*, **15**, 198-201.

Fink, S. L., Skipper, J. K. and Hallenbeck, P. N. (1968). Physical disability and problems in marriage. *J. Marr. Family*, **30**, 64-73.

Fisher, S. (1973). *The Female Orgasm*, Allen Lane, New York.

Fitzpatrick, W. F. (1972). Sexual function in the paraplegic patient. *Arch. phys. Med. Rehab.*, **55**, 221-227.

Francois, N., Lichtenberger, J.-M., Jonannet, P., Desert, J.-F. and Manry, M. (1980). L'éjaculation par de vibro-massage chez le paraplégique à propos de 50 cas avec 7 grosses. *Ann. Méd. phys.*, **23**, 24-36.

Gillan, P. and Brindley, G. S. (1979). Vaginal and pelvic floor responses to sexual stimulation. *Psychophysiology*, **16**, 471-481.

Griffith, E. R., Tomke, M. A. and Timms, R. J. (1973). Sexual function in spinal cord injury patients: a review. *Arch. phys. Med. Rehab.*, **54**, 514-543.

Guttman, W. L. (1964). Married life of paraplegics and tetraplegics. *Paraplegia*, **2**, 182-188.

Horne, H. W., Paull, D. P. and Munro, D. (1948). Fertility studies in human male with traumatic injuries of the spinal cord and cauda equina. *New Engl. J. Med.*, **239**, 959-961.

Kaplan, H. S. (1974). *The New Sex Therapy*, Brunner/Mazel, New York.

Kiesler, A., Collins, C. and Miller, M. (1969). *Attitude Change*, Wiley, New York.

Kinsey, A. C., Pomeroy, W. B., Martin, E. C. and Gebhard, P. M. (1953). *Sexual Behaviour in the Human Female*, Saunders, Philadelphia.

Langevin, R. and Martin, M. (1975). Can erotic responses be classically conditioned? *Behav. Ther.*, 6, 350-356.

Laughren, T. P. and Kass, D. J. (1975). Desensitization of sexual dysfunction: the present status. In *Couples in Conflict* (Ed. A. S. Gurman and D. G. Rice), Aronson, New York.

Lobitz, W. C. and Lo Piccolo, J. (1972). New methods in the behavioural treatment of sexual dysfunction. *J. Behav. Ther. exptl Psychiat.*, 3, 265-271.

Masters, W. H. and Johnson, V. E. (1966). *Human Sexual Responses*, Little Brown, Boston.

Masters, W. H. and Johnson, V. E. (1970). *Human Sexual Inadequacy*, Little Brown, Boston.

Paintin, D. B. (1976). The physiology of sex. In *Psychosexual Problems* (Ed. H. Milne and S. J. Hardy), Bradford Press, London.

Teal, J. C. and Atheston, G. T. (1975). Sexuality and spinal cord injury: Some psychosocial considerations. *Arch. phys. Med. Rehab.*, 56, 264-268.

Wincze, J. P. and Caird, W. K. (1976). The effects of systematic desensitization and video desensitization in the treatment of essential sexual dysfunction in woman. *Behav. Ther.*, 7, 335-342.

Zeitlin, A. B., Cottrell, T. L. and Lloyd, F. A. (1957). Sexology of the paraplegic male. *Fertil. Steril.*, 8, 337-344.

8. The role of the Disablement Resettlement Officer

Derek Willcocks

Over the past 30 years the government employment policies for disabled people have been based on the principle that, given the right sort of support services, most disabled people can compete for jobs on equal terms with anyone else. The Manpower Services Commission (MSC) feels that this principle is still valid today. The provision of specialised services for disabled people is a very important part of the Manpower Services Commission's work, and a substantial share of its resources is devoted to this field.

It is often forgotten that most disabled people who are able to work are actually in employment. Even so, extra support needs to be available for those who are unemployed. The MSC therefore aims to continue to provide, maintain and indeed improve the services necessary to help disabled people to choose, train for, obtain and keep worth-while jobs. To reinforce the point that this part of the work is a priority area, no reduction was made in the staffing or the resources allocated in 1982 to the resettlement services for the disabled, despite quite substantial staff cuts that have been made in the MSC as a whole.

The MSC provides help for the disabled through a national network of Jobcentres, through the MSC's training services and Youth Opportunity Programme, through the provision of special schemes and aids to employment, through the Fit For Work Award Scheme, and through the provision of employment rehabilitation and the sheltered employment programme. In 1980/81 £115 million was spent, over 13 per cent of the MSC budget, assisting disabled people. More than 2600 staff deal solely with the disabled.

These efforts resulted in work for almost 40 000 disabled people in 1980/81 operational year, plus an estimated further 6000 job placements for disabled people who used what is referred to as the self-service section of Jobcentres. During the same year more than 16 000 people undertook assessment courses at Employment Rehabilitation Centres; 4000 disabled people completed training courses for open employment; nearly 14 000 severely disabled people were being employed in sheltered industry; and some 4000 special aids were on permanent loan to disabled people at work.

RETURN TO WORK

The work of the MSC will not normally begin until clients are well on the way to recovery from their injury and coming round the final bend of the road back to employment. Employment is the Manpower Services Commission's business. It aims to serve people who, because of disability or the residual effects of illness, will need extra help to find or to return to employment.

The cornerstone, the linch-pin, of all the work in this field is the Disablement Resettlement Officer (DRO). The DRO, trained to help disabled people find work, can be a patient's passport to the wide range of specialist services which the MSC provides to help disabled people to find and keep employment (see figure 8.1).

A DRO is based in most of the larger Job Centres. There are about 500 on the UK mainland, including more than 70 in the Greater London area.

Services and schemes which the DRO can suggest or recommend to help the disabled to find and keep employment can be grouped into four main areas.

(1) Preparation for work: (a) employment rehabilitation, (b) training, (c) Youth Opportunities Programme.

(2) Help with job finding: (a) self-service, (b) specialist advice and placing, (c) job introduction scheme.

(3) At work: (a) fares to work, (b) special aids, (c) adaptations to premises.

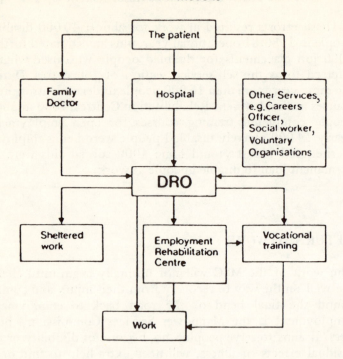

Figure 8.1 The role of the Disablement Resettlement Officer.

(4) Sheltered employment: (a) sheltered workshops, (b) sheltered industrial groups, (c) homeworkers' schemes, (d) business on own account.

Details of these main areas are as follows.

Preparation for work

Employment rehabilitation

The Commission provides special courses at Employment Rehabilitation Centres (ERCs) for those who have been ill, injured or unemployed for some time. The courses are designed to increase confidence and motivation, to give vocational guidance and assessment in preparation for work or training. As far as is practicable, the ERCs are organised along the lines of a factory or office, in order to create a realistic working atmosphere. Much of the output consists of actual production work obtained from local firms or government departments.

The DRO liaises closely with ERC staff in individual resettlement cases and most applications for rehabilitation courses are routed through him. He gives special attention to the placing of ex-rehabilitees. The ERC is often the first stage in an individual resettlement plan. It may be followed either directly by employment, possibly using job rehearsal, or by a period of training. Job rehearsal allows a client to spend up to 6 weeks on an actual job while still in receipt of rehabilitation allowances. Clients are not always referred from hospital. Any doctor may refer a client direct to the resident doctor at an ERC for an assessment.

Training

Most disabled people are able to benefit from general training opportunities scheme (TOPS) courses, of which there are now over 600. The eligibility conditions are less stringent for disabled people — for example, admission to training can be at any time after school-leaving age and a second course may be given in less than 3 years. Four *residential training colleges* (RTCs) cater for the needs of the more severely handicapped, while the special *Individual Training Throughout with an Employer* (ITTWE) scheme for disabled people offers sponsored training on an employer's premises for up to a year or more, followed by employment.

Youth Opportunities Programme

Young disabled people can take advantage of opportunities for work preparation and work experience under the MSC's Special Programmes Division, where, again, the eligibility conditions are relaxed. For example, a Young Person's Work Preparation Course could be arranged. This is a special 13 week course run at an Employment Rehabilitation Centre, designed to give young people a chance to try out lots of different kinds of work to see which is most suitable for the individual client. During the course help will be given on such topics as applying for jobs, how to cope with job interviews, wages, and many other aspects needed every day at work.

Alternatively, the client might benefit from a period of work experience in one of a number of locations. For example, with a company, in a workshop or with a community group, in order to get first-hand experience of real work.

The MSC's training and Youth Opportunity Programmes are currently being reorganised and integrated into a comprehensive £1 billion youth training scheme, which is planned to start in September 1983. The needs of disabled people will continue to be taken fully into account.

Help with job finding

Self-service

Assistance to disabled people and their employers is available as an integral part of the general employment service in Jobcentres. Indeed, the policy is to encourage this wherever possible. As a result, many disabled people are placed, unidentified, through self-service each year. Encouraging disabled people to use self-service allows more time for the DRO to spend with those in more need of help and advice.

Specialist advice and placing

This area of activity is at the core of the MSC's Resettlement Service, and is very much the prerogative of the DRO. Of the 500 local office DROs, the majority are peripatetic and a small number are outstationed full-time at selected large hospitals. There is also an Assistant DRO at every local office to give placing and clerical support to the DRO. There are 35 specially trained Blind Persons Resettlement Officers who provide a specialist service for blind and partially sighted people.

In broad terms, the work of Disablement Resettlement Officers is to encourage employers to take on disabled people and to help them find jobs they can do well and which give satisfaction. At the same time, DROs have to ensure that disabled people make the best use of the services available to them.

DROs can draw on expert advice provided as required by hospitals, general practitioners, regional medical services or specialists from the Employment Medical Advisory Service. With help of this kind to reinforce their own skills, DROs are able to assess the type of work that is likely to be most suitable and congenial to individual disabled people. Through close contacts with employers they know what job opportunities are available and, most important, they have a sound knowledge of what is needed to do each job effectively, so that an employer can be confident that if the DRO recommends someone for a particular job, that applicant is capable of doing it.

Another increasingly important aspect of the DRO's work at a time when redundancies are occurring is to give employers advice on the retention of disabled workers. This might involve restructuring the job, retraining or the use of special aids.

Job Introduction Scheme

Under this scheme, introduced exclusively for disabled people, employers may be given a weekly grant towards the cost of the trial period for a disabled job-seeker. Experience has shown that in many cases the employer offers the disabled person a permanent job at the end of the trial period.

At work

Fares to work

Assistance towards the costs of fares to and from work can be given to disabled people if they are unable to use public transport for their journey because of their disability. Under this scheme a weekly cash grant can be paid.

Special aids to employment

The MSC issues on free permanent loan any special tools or equipment which a disabled person needs to enable him or her to obtain or keep employment. Many of the aids are loaned to blind and partially sighted people. Examples include closed circuit television, talking calculators, brailled measuring equipment, Optacon reading machines, tape recorders and braille computer terminals.

Sighted disabled people often need individual solutions to their particular employment problems. These may include special-purpose jigs and fixtures; special fitments for tools; purpose-built desks, seats and benches; counter-balanced drawing boards and tilting stands and tables; electric typewriters; telephone aids and accessories; and reading and writing aids.

DROs call upon the services of technical officers to give advice on the most suitable personal aid to solve employment difficulties.

Adaptations to premises

Some disabled people have difficulty climbing steps or getting into the toilet at work. Others might require some modification to a piece of machinery to make it easier to operate. These difficulties can be overcome by employers making use of the MSC's Adaptations to Premises and Equipment scheme.

Grants of up to £6000 may be paid to employers who need to adapt their premises or equipment to enable them to recruit or retain in employment a specified disabled person. It may be that a ramp is required to enable access to be gained to a place of employment or a toilet might need to be adapted. Grants can be made towards the cost of these types of adaptations.

Sheltered employment

It is the DRO's responsibility to identify those people who are so seriously disabled that they are unlikely to be capable of work other than under sheltered conditions and to try to place them into sheltered employment. These people may be helped through:

(a) *Sheltered workshops* — operated by Remploy (as the statutory body), local authorities and voluntary organisations with financial support from MSC.

(b) *Sheltered industrial groups* — small groups of severely disabled people working under special supervision in normal industry and commerce, sponsored by a 'parent' organisation, which may be either a local authority or a voluntary organisation. The DRO has an important role to play in identifying opportunities for setting up sheltered industrial groups.

(c) *Homeworkers' schemes* - homework centres are based on Remploy factories and provide work for people who are homebound owing to disability. Workers are paid piecework rates. Other schemes are sponsored by local authorities and supported by MSC grants.

(d) *Business on own account* — grants can be made available to enable severely disabled people to set up their own business.

DRO REFERRALS

There are three main sources from which the DRO builds up his clientele case load:

(1) Registrants and other callers (self-referrals).

(2) Referrals from doctors, hospitals, social services, voluntary organisations, employers.

(3) DRO visits and contacts.

The DRO will arrange the initial interview at the local Jobcentre if the disabled person is able to attend. If not, the DRO will arrange to call at the client's home or visit him or her in hospital.

Members of the rehabilitation team have a very important role to play in helping the DRO to make full use of employment opportunities for disabled people. They need to identify and advise the DRO of cases where a return to work, or retraining for another job, would benefit a client. The earlier the referral is made the better the opportunity for rehabilitation. If the DRO is able to draw up a resettlement plan for a patient before medical care ends, the return to work is part of a continuous rehabilitation programme. This is preferable to having a gap in the process during which time the patient may well lose confidence and motivation.

APPENDIX

Further details of the services and schemes mentioned above are contained in the following leaflets, which are available free at Jobcentres and Employment Offices:

Employing disabled people	(EPL 61)
Employing someone who is deaf or hard of hearing	(EPL 38)
Employing someone with epilepsy	(EPL 40)
Employing someone who is mentally handicapped	(EPL 44)
Employing someone who is blind or partially sighted	(EPL 63)
Employing people who have had a mental illness	(EPL 93)
Employing someone with haemophilia	(EPL 98)
Employing someone with multiple sclerosis	(EPL 102)
Assistance with Fares to Work Scheme for severely disabled people	(DPL 13)
Employment Rehabilitation Centres	(EPL 30)
Aids and adaptations for disabled employees	(EPL 71)
Job introduction for disabled people	(DPL 15)
All that counts is ability	(TSD L109)
Train for a better job with TOPS	(TSD N100)
Training opportunities for disabled people	(TSD N127)
Fit for Work Award Scheme	(ESP 69)
Employment in sheltered workshops	(DPL 11)
Sheltered industrial groups	(EPL 95)
Sheltered employment and you	(EPL 99)
The Disabled Persons (Employment) Acts 1944 and 1958	(DPL 2)

9. Help in the community

Michael Smith and Ann Macfarlane

The role of community physicians is to seek out and give advice on the health care of the population they are appointed to serve. Although community physicians are doctors who specialise in preventive medicine, they rarely, if ever, see individual patients, but their influence in the community can be considerable. They tend to specialise in child health, social services and environmental health.

If there is a doctor in an area who has the title Specialist in Community Medicine (Social Services), he can be approached for help to provide better care for all physically handicapped — not just paraplegics. He can assist in the following ways:

(1) Help to initiate within each health authority the establishment of a Specialist Joint Care Planning Team (JCPT) especially for the physically disabled. These officially appointed teams can comprise those people with a special interest who are members of the health authority, local interested groups, and officers of the health and local authorities. They should have a subject expertise that is the best that is locally available.

(2) Seek support through the Specialist JCPT for money from the joint finance allocation, which, incidentally, is the only finance for health service which has actually increased in recent years in England and Wales as a whole. The priorities for the use of this separate allocation have to be jointly agreed (hence the name) between local and health authorities. The spending of it is then sanctioned by the health authority.

(3) A community physician may be approached to liaise informally between local or national interest groups and the professions. This is one of the most fruitful ways for patient groups to feed in new ideas and to receive whatever health service support can be forthcoming.

Finance available to the National Health Service has been reduced, particularly in the south of England. In difficult times it is our experience that the proselytisers do best. The community physician, once convinced of the case to be made for specific resources for the handicapped, can be a powerful proselytiser.

In the case of the handicapped — who are an NHS priority group — their real needs can be supported in their claim to NHS resources, so it is important to establish contact with the local community physician.

It cannot be stressed too frequently how important is the team effort of the physiotherapist, occupational therapist and social worker, whose communication and liaison with the paraplegic and the family is vital if the transition from hospital to home life is to be as painless as possible.

Previous chapters have looked at their work in assessing the patient and making recommendations for alterations and adaptations to homes, but for most disabled people the key to overcoming their disability lies in one which will fit the door of an adapted or purpose-built house or flat. Most conventional homes have some inconvenience in their design which for the able-bodied can be tolerated, but the disabled person must be critical for their independence if they are to carry out personal and household tasks. What are the possibilities? A knowledge of the different types of housing for the disabled is essential.

TYPES OF HOUSING

Wheelchair housing

Wheelchair housing — probably the most suitable for the paraplegic — is specially planned for people confined to wheelchairs and the important feature is generous spacing for wheelchair manoeuvre. In a new housing complex a few units should be incorporated to allow for integration in the community.

The dwelling should be situated where there is ease of access to the community facilities such as shops, library, post office, church or place of work. Important features in the design are:

(a) A level or slightly ramped approach to the entrance, with no threshold obstruction.

(b) Internal space for wheelchair manoeuvre. Passageways should be 1200 mm wide, fitted with suitable doors. Sliding doors should have a 2 ft 6½ in opening and all doors should have easy-to-reach grab handles for closing.

(c) A kitchen planned with sufficient space to turn the wheelchair and with access to equipment and storage units. The height of work surfaces, electrical appliances and cupboards and drawers is crucial to the independence of the wheelchair user. Individuals will have varying requirements but attention to detail is essential. A separate oven and hob unit is a 'must' for the disabled, with free space under each unit. A mirror positioned over the hob will enable contents of saucepans to be viewed while cooking. 'D' handles on doors and cupboards are helpful for those with weak hands. A gadget can be obtained to assist with turning conventional or lever taps.

(d) A bathroom planned for wheelchair use should have sufficient space to transfer to bath or shower.

(e) A toilet designed for transfer from a wheelchair.

(f) Fitments such as light switches, electrical sockets and window catches should be placed at a height suitable for wheelchair users.

(g) Large windows, placed to give maximum light and views.

(h) A garage or carport, with undercover access to the dwelling.

(i) A central heating system which is flexible and economic. It is important for the paraplegic to maintain an even body temperature, and the central heating controls should be suitably positioned for easy adjustment.

Mobility housing

It may be possible for wheelchair users to be accommodated in mobility housing units. Basically, this type of housing has

no steps or stairs and can take the form of (a) a bungalow;
(b) a ground-floor flat; (c) a flat on an upper level serviced by
a lift; (d) a house with a bathroom and a bedroom at ground
level; (e) a two-storey house incorporating a lift operating
between the living room and bedroom, or which has a straight
staircase to which a stairlift can be fitted.

Mobility housing may not be ideal for the wheelchair user
but it may help to alleviate the effect of disability until
wheelchair housing becomes available.

Housing adaptations

A family home may be difficult or impossible for the paraplegic or tetraplegic to run, but it may not be practicable or
desirable for the family to move to a more spacious or
specially designed dwelling. So many factors have to be
considered by the newly disabled person, including the cost
of erecting a purpose-built dwelling, which may be prohibi-
tive. It may be that the most practicable solution will be to
adapt the existing dwelling, and these adaptations can be
approved and carried out by the local authority.

They could include: (a) a ramp or ramps to improve
wheelchair access; (b) the installation of a lift or stair-lift;
(c) the substitution of a shower for a bath; (d) alterations to
an existing toilet or a ground-floor toilet installed; (e) alterations to the kitchen; (f) if space permits, the addition of a
bedroom and bathroom on the ground floor.

The social services authority is obliged by law to arrange
for an adaptation to be made where necessary. The authority
is not obliged to pay for or undertake the work. The Department of the Environment, Department of Health and Social
Security and the Welsh Office (Circular DofE 59/78) advise
that for adaptations to housing association and council
property housing authorities should be responsible for
funding structural adaptations, and social services should
undertake payment for equipment and aids (see Chapters 5
and 6). The term 'structural' may mean any work for which a
building contractor may be employed. While a stair-lift and
hoist installation may be funded directly by the local authority

or housing association, these adaptations may be treated as a social services responsibility. For owner-occupiers or privately rented property the initial approach made by, or on behalf of, the disabled person to the social worker, the occupational therapist or housing officer, may be followed by a recommendation to apply for an intermediate or improvement grant. Contact will then need to be made with the officer in the district council responsible for grants, who will usually be in the environmental health department.

As a general rule, under the terms of the 1974 and 1980 Housing Acts, all owner-occupiers and tenants are entitled to apply for grants.

GRANTS

Two forms of grant are available to help the disabled person (see Chapter 6).

(1) *Improvement grant.* This grant is for structural work needed to make a dwelling suitable for the accommodation, welfare or employment of a disabled person where the existing building is inadequate or unsuitable. It is important to remember that equipment and aids are the responsibility of the social services department.

(2) *Intermediate grant.* This grant is for the provision of additional standard amenities for the use of the disabled occupant, such as bath, toilet, basin and sink. Improvement grants are made at the discretion of the local authority, but intermediate grants are mandatory, which means that the local authority must make a grant, provided that it is satisfied that existing standard amenities are not readily accessible to the disabled occupant by reason of his disability. For example, it may be that the existing toilet is on the first floor and the disabled person cannot climb the stairs. The amount of the grant is based on the cost of the work approved for grant. This is called the eligible expense and is subject to a limit. The grant is a percentage of the eligible expense. Eligible expense limits are higher in London than elsewhere in England and Wales.

For both kinds of grant the rate in priority cases is 75 per cent of the cost of the work, and this can be increased to 90 per cent in cases of financial hardship.

It is important to realise that wheelchair and mobility housing does exist, although in short supply, and that financial help can be obtained to adapt existing accommodation.

TRANSPORT

It is not sufficient to leave the paraplegic with an accessible home environment. To lead an active life mobility outside the home is needed. Advice will have been given to the patient while in hospital (see Chapter 5).

Transport is vital if a return to work, or retraining, is envisaged, and for the paraplegic this is essential, as he is likely to live a normal life-span and will need usefully to occupy his time. Where a paraplegic has received a large sum of money in compensation for his accident or injury, there may be less incentive to work. Good counselling is necessary to ensure wise use of resources, but where a paraplegic is able to purchase or adapt an existing car, it is likely that he, or she, will be entitled to the Mobility Allowance, which is non-taxable. To qualify for this the age limit is 5–66. The allowance may be spent in any way but it is intended to be for outdoor mobility. It is not means-tested, and an applicant must be unable, or virtually unable, to walk and likely to remain so for at least a year. Leaflet NI 225 explains how to claim the Mobility Allowance.

A voluntary organisation, Motability, was set up on the initiative of the Government to help disabled people get maximum benefit from the Mobility Allowance to acquire a car. It offers a leasing and hire purchase scheme and full details can be obtained from Motability at Boundary House, London (see Appendix 1).

People with severe disabilities, who cannot drive a car, may be entitled to help with fares to and from work from the Manpower Services Commission (see Chapter 8).

In some areas 'Dial-a-Ride' transport is available. This is

run like a taxi service and is useful if a person is unable to drive or is awaiting an adapted vehicle.

Some voluntary organisations own vehicles with tail-lifts and use them for transporting their members to meetings. These may be loaned for other purposes, such as taking a disabled person on holiday.

Travel by air is probably one of the easiest forms of transport, and the airport authorities issue booklets on help that can be expected if details of a disabled person's needs are made prior to the flight date.

British Rail operate a rail-card scheme for the disabled, and a card can be purchased for £10 per annum. This allows travel with an escort by paying one second-class fare. Ferry and hovercraft operators are also aware of the needs of the disabled traveller. Coach steps are difficult to negotiate, but if a person is able to be lifted up the steps by able helpers, then coach firms will readily help.

CONCLUSION

For the paraplegic there is a bewildering maze of agencies willing to try to assist in the home and in the community. So many things previously taken for granted have to be seriously considered — where to live, how to be as mobile as possible, where to shop, how to cope with the housework, what work to do, where to spend a holiday and how to locate accessible toilets on a journey. The paraphernalia connected with daily living can be daunting and exhausting, but if the right information is available, trauma can be reduced. In some parts of the UK there are associations which run advisory services for the disabled and their relatives. The Citizens Advice Bureau can give local information on these. Other useful contacts are listed at the end of this book.

REFERENCES

DHSS Leaflet NI 225: *Mobility Allowance.*
DofE Circular 59/78: *Adaptations to Housing Association and Council Property.*

10. Living a normal life

Tim Marshall

Recovering from serious injury, the patient needs to consider a number of aspects and tries to look at his or her own situation objectively. Previous chapters have looked at housing, employment and the need to respect family circumstances, but the possible extent of the patient's objectivity is both limited and conditioned by personal experience. From within the highly organised and structured hospital day the patient peers forward into something of a haze, wondering how whatever arrangements have been made will work out. Some will work but, as with life in general, probably some will not, and coping with such uncertainty, successfully or otherwise, is called living.

ASPECTS OF REHABILITATION

The patient needs to look at aspects of the social and psychological background to rehabilitation against which 'the basics' for living a normal life need to be viewed. Rehabilitation can be defined as the process of learning to live with one's own disability in one's own environment. Traditionally, this has consisted of teaching people to learn to perform physical aids to daily living and self-care skills, and success in these has been regarded as evidence of good rehabilitation.

'But', asks Trieschmann (1980), 'are physical skills the appropriate criteria of success in rehabilitation?

'Does the ability to transfer in and out of a wheelchair, or to groom oneself, ensure success in coping with the world as a disabled person? The abilities to walk and groom oneself do not ensure success in the able-bodied person, since these are tasks that are mastered by the age of five to seven years in most persons. After mastering these physical tasks life consists of learning to interact with other people and the environment in order to gain some degree of satisfaction.'

It may be an unfair comparison that children have another 10–15 years in which 'society' allows them to interact with other people before being granted 'adult' status and being expected to behave in an 'adult' way, whereas spinal cord injury cases have at most a few months in an initially highly stressful and always highly artificial environment to learn, or relearn, such interacting skills.

It is worth considering why such learning, or relearning, is necessary at all. According to Trieschmann: 'The concept of difference is learned at an early age, as is the concept of physical attractiveness, and we learn to evaluate people on these two dimensions. Thus the person with spinal injury may devalue himself according to these standards that he himself learned and he knows that others will devalue him accordingly. As a result, the person with spinal injury tends to withdraw from most social situations after discharge from the rehabilitation center.' Goffmann (1963) offers a similar argument: 'The painfulness, then, of sudden stigmatisation can come not from the individual's confusion about his identity, but from his knowing too well what he has become.'

Self-perceived devaluation, however, is not all, nor often as extensive as is thought. The 'others' mentioned by Trieschmann may even include rehabilitation staff themselves. Taylor (1967) asked staff and new patients to complete a psychological questionnaire in a manner describing the reactions of a newly injured person with spinal cord injury. The findings showed that the staff had no real understanding of what these reactions were really like. They consistently over-estimated the degree of psychological stress and depression, and reflected very much the negative stereotype of the disabled person. As Lawson (1977) has pointed out, many disabled persons report that the most depressing thing about being a patient is that the staff expect them to be depressed.

Life *does* consist of interacting with others, and to an extent the satisfaction gained depends on the expectations we have of each other and of ourselves. It is almost too easy to abandon the sort of relationships and life style to which one was accustomed before an injury, and to settle into fulfilling one's own and others' stereotyped expectations of what the 'disabled person' does, or can do. The avoidance of this, by a positive seeking out and grasping of wider opportunities, is important.

As has been said earlier, the three essential factors necessary to living a normal life are: somewhere to live, some way of getting about, and something to do. These three factors are like a tripod — if one leg is taken away, the 'whole thing' collapses. One-word summaries of these three factors come down to housing, mobility and employment/occupation, and in one form or another they have all been covered earlier in the book. Trieschmann has a similar although not identical triad associated with living a successful ('normal') life, whether or not the person is disabled: the prevention of medical complications and the utilisation of ADL (activities of daily living) and mobility skills; the maintenance of a stable living environment; and 'productivity' (which may or may not involve employment). We overlap to a considerable extent. If anything, my emphasis is on the 'hardware' — a house, a car, a job — whereas Trieschmann's is on the 'software' — the successful operation and management of whatever hardware is available.

WORK

With regard to 'work', we have to recognise that employment, or self-employment, is not necessarily an appropriate goal for everyone to aim at. Fallon (1979) puts this point particularly well with the bald question, 'Why do you want to work?' In truth, not all will need to, for the prospect of a large capital sum in compensation for injury, or a lifetime service or industrial pension, may appear to offer financial security, for which, of course, most people have to work. Nevertheless, there will still be a need to do something on discharge, for even the most severely injured people find that daily self-care activities, whether they are able to manage by themselves or need help, simply do not fill up the whole day.

The range of what is possible, or suitable, will, of course, depend enormously on the individual and his or her circumstances. Post-discharge 'activity' is something which can hardly be discussed too early, and post-injury counselling about this ought to encompass the notion that economic productivity is not the only possible goal. Where it is, in many cases, the most useful channel of advice about employment will be via the DRO or the Housing Rehabilitation Officer, if one exists. A few people will be fortunate enough to be assured of re-employment by their previous employer, and, provided that the job itself is not a downgrading from the former one, any such offer should be grasped with both hands. It is as near a return to the previous normality as will be possible.

Arguments can be heard on both sides about whether or not to accept a job below the previous level of qualification, and practical considerations may eventually dictate what one does. In accepting a lesser job there is the risk of being devalued by others as to one's capabilities and ultimately of lowering one's own expectations accordingly.

Similar considerations affect applying for a job in the first place, and there is an interesting divergence of opinion noted by Fallon as to whether a potential employer should be informed about the use of a wheelchair at the application stage. 'Professionals', she says, 'advise yes'; but many disabled people, with the hindsight of experience, have concluded that to do so invites rejection without a proper consideration of the applicant's qualifications. This is probably an example of employers either undervaluing people with spinal cord injury, or simply not wanting to be involved with anything they imagine might be a troublesome, or possibly embarrassing, experience. From the disabled side, there is a determination not to be put at a potential disadvantage until absolutely unavoidable − by which time there will be the opportunity to convince an employer face to face of one's abilities.

Retraining or acquiring academic qualifications will be a necessary route for some, and this is likely to open up other previously closed avenues. But, of course, not everyone will either want, or be capable of, this. It is not possible to push everyone to worldly success on the escalator of education. There is a wide range of 'things to do' beyond the realms of employment and education to which some people will need

126   *Tim Marshall*

to be introduced while they are in hospital. The tasks of disabled people, according to Gunn and Peterson (1978): '. . . have been to acquire a job, attain acceptance by "normal" people, and achieve functional levels of behaviour. Little effort has been exerted to assist this group to achieve the socio-leisure skills so essential to the rest of the culture. Yet, if there was ever a group who needed a release from tensions and problems and who needed to find ways for self-development and expression, social interaction, relaxation, mastering of skills, and just plain fun, it is the disabled.' The case for teaching newly disabled people how to find 'something to do' cannot be less strong than this.

THE VOLUNTARY SOCIETY

Voluntary societies seem to be expanding exponentially, in number if not in size, and everywhere one turns there seems to be another group of people starting an organisation and inviting one to join. They range from local, geographically based organisations through activity-specific clubs, especially sports clubs (the *Society of One-armed Golfers*) to disability-specific societies such as the *Spinal Injuries Association* (SIA).

Perhaps the first question to ask is whether an association such as the SIA can help while one is in hospital, and if so, how. There is no doubt from talking to 'old' spinal cord injury people there appears to be considerable psychotherapeutic value in meeting members of the Association, whether as in-patients or as out-patients. The impression gained is that these are just normal people, leading ordinary lives, and therefore so can you (see Fallon, 1976).

The *'Link'* scheme, where 'A. Para ("old-established")' is put in touch with a new case (if the latter wishes) from the same locality, in similar circumstances – age, sex, family situation, and so on –, is something which only a voluntary organisation can undertake. In its way it is an informal attempt at peer counselling, and although I know of no formal, rigorous evaluation of the scheme, anecdotal evidence suggests that it is very much welcomed by some, and probably doesn't do much harm to any others – one can, after all, refuse to have anything to do with it!

It is after discharge that the voluntary organisation can come into its own. The fact that the counselling service established by the SIA is, to say the least, heavily used suggests that many people do not feel able to use the statutory medical or social services to solve some of the problems related to their disability, or that they have failed to obtain satisfactory help. Apart from individual casework, there are situations which only a voluntary organisation is in a position to exploit, and there is a diversity of information relevant to the condition which it would be most unusual, if not impossible, for the ordinary individual to encounter in the course of everyday life.

A few examples should illustrate this diversity.

It was following a campaign by the Spinal Injuries Association that the company Everest and Jennings (subsequently Zimmer, and now Carters) were once again allowed to issue their wheelchairs to 'young, active' disabled people after the withdrawal of this facility in the early 1970s on grounds of cost.

It was a campaign by the SIA, including the most detailed exposition to ministers and civil servants by its chairman, Lady Masham, which finally brought safe, non-splitting plastics 'Disposa-gloves' on to the drug tariff.

SIA was not alone in either of these campaigns, but played a major part in their development, where certainly the paraplegic person, as an individual, could have had little effect.

All-age driving licences are another achievement of the organisation on behalf of people specifically with spinal cord injury, following an initial breakthrough by an individual member in a court case. Here the SIA even managed to extract an admission that the belief of consultants in the inadvisability of issuing all-age driving licences was in fact no more than a belief, and there was no medical evidence to support it.

These three examples all appeared in the SIA newsletter, as did detailed explanations of how to arrange for artificial

insemination by donor (AID) or artificial insemination by
husband (AIH). This kind of specialised information is
unlikely to be found through the media, and possibly, even
today, is something that some general practitioners might
not be aware of.

Information ranging from a rebate on the first 4 years of
Mobility Allowance payments to which hotels to stay at can
be obtained from voluntary organisations. It is this mixture,
together with the weight they can bring to bear on particular
issues, which makes them so valuable.

RECREATION AND LEISURE

There is plenty of leisure time in the first few weeks in hospital. The patient cannot go anywhere, except when pushed
by someone else. Little exercise is possible, except working
springs and slings hung around the cage attached to the bed.
Despite eating, being washed and turned, and ward rounds,
there is a huge amount of time for which the options seem to
be talking and listening, reading or writing, perhaps painting,
and sleeping. There is little chance of pursuing actively any
new leisure interests, unless the patient fancies writing the
definite exposé of life in an acute unit, but it has been done
so many times already. The weekly film is an entertainment,
a high spot – at any rate, something *different* from the
television.

Need it be so? I think not – although, to judge from my
own experience in hospital, there was little attempt during
the first 3 months to interest people in anything which might
have become a recreation later on. Admitting that the resources
of the hospital do not extend to employing people to arrange
different types of activity, it seems to me that potential
resources in the community are all but ignored. For example,
a talk given by the local photographic club, the local music
society or the pigeon fanciers' club might be of interest.
Something on these lines would be worth trying, although it
would need to be very carefully evaluated.

Once the patient begins getting up, the range of options
widens enormously. Recreational therapy is the name of the

game in the USA. Although judgement should be reserved about some of the more expansive claims made for it, the principle of offering to new spinal cord injury cases a wide range of activities in order to provoke or develop new recreational interests, which may eventually become lifetime recreational pursuits, seems excellent. Drama, music and art therapy are all offered on a regular basis in some hospitals, together with the ubiquitous sport.

Sport is sometimes seen as a panacea for everything. It is difficult to avoid it in a spinal injury unit, even though no one is forced to take part, for all the most successful disabled sports clubs are based on these units. Not so in America, where clubs tend to be much more sport-specific, and community- rather than hospital-based. In the UK there is a fairly narrow range of activities to which the new spinal cord injury case will be exposed while in hospital, and the model of successful sporting achievement will be that outlined in Guttmann's book *Textbook of Sport for the Disabled*.

I have become less keen on this approach, not because I do not approve of sport, but because it offers too narrow a view of what is possible — sailing, canoeing, subaqua, water skiing, winter sports — all offered within a virtually segregated setting. For more examples see Norman Croucher's book *Outdoor Pursuits for Disabled People*. If a paraplegic wants to play basketball, then it must be with other people in wheelchairs, but why should there not be wheelchair sections to the *able-bodied* basketball clubs, in the same way that there are women's and youth's sections? This would also apply to track and field athletics.

One of the problems of organising sporting, or other, activities in a segregated setting is that it comes to be seen by the rest of the world as the natural order of things for people in wheelchairs to play, compete and associate with other people in wheelchairs. This is, I think, less an active form of reasoning than simply an interpretation of what appears to happen. It does indeed seem that people with disabilities are often content to develop social circles consisting mainly of other people in wheelchairs. It is, however, inconsistent to complain that the rest of the world behaves towards you in a stereotyped fashion if, by your own actions, you demonstrate an apparent wish for social segregation.

In one sense this is an extreme view, and therefore likely to be unpopular. There are good reasons for people with spinal cord injury to get together in an organisation to press for the types of services and facilities outlined earlier. There is, however, an almost invisible but crucially important line between aggregation for these purposes (and whatever social relationships may evolve as a result) and the deliberate aggregation of people with spinal cord injury primarily for mutual social support. This latter form of socialisation is probably very necessary for some, possibly many, people, but it is a pity that it is so. It indicates a lack of social reintegration which should have been accomplished by the time someone leaves hospital.

There is a passage from Ann Shearer's recent book, *Disability — Whose Handicap?*, which is obliquely relevant to this situation, and is worth quoting. It concerns the residential segregation of people with particular disabilities.

' "People who are blind and mute", said the Massachusetts Board of State Charities, "often exhibit morbid tendencies.

"Now these are lessened, and their morbid effects corrected in each individual, by intimate intercourse with persons of good and normal condition — that is, by general society; while they are strengthened by associating closely and persistently with others having the like infirmity. . . . Guided by this principle, we should, in providing for the instruction and training of these persons, have the association among them as little as possible, and counteract its tendencies by encouraging association and intimacy with common society. They should be kept together no more closely and no longer than necessary for their special instruction; and there should be no attempt to build up permanent asylums for them, or to favour the establishment of communities composed wholly, or mainly of persons subject to a common infirmity".'

The principles of non-segregation outlined in that passage should extend to virtually all areas of life — particularly in work and leisure. What is remarkable about it is that it was written in 1866!

Recreation and leisure activities can consist of whatever a disabled person wants to do, provided that they have the confidence to contact and persuade clubs, organisations and individuals to give them the opportunity to compete. A considerable degree of perseverance will probably be needed to convince such people of their abilities, but if they persist, the rewards of broader social contact will be there. The disabled need encouragement to 'get on and be yourself' and not to be the disabled stereotype.

CONCLUSION

Trieschmann has wise words to say about how this is to be accomplished: 'Basically the emphasis in rehabilitation should shift from physical functioning to psycho-social integration into the community. The latter entails the former, but the reverse is not true.' We need, in hospital, to equip people with the social confidence to pursue occupational and recreational goals limited only by their wishes, and not by the test of social rejection. The goal to be aimed at, that of including disabled people fully in society, is summed up in the following passage from a conference held in Texas in 1980: 'The concept of inclusion implies a fundamentally new definition of handicapped persons, not as people who are "less than complete" but as full members of society with the rights and responsibilities of all citizens. Inclusion is not based on pity, compassion, charity or fear. Rather, it stems from a humanist belief in the fundamental importance of the ability, self-determination, dignity and worth of all persons'.

REFERENCES

Croucher, N. (1981). *Outdoor Pursuits for Disabled People*, Disabled Living Foundation, London.
Fallon, B. (1976). *So You're Paralysed. . .* , Spinal Injuries Association, London.
Fallon, B. (1979). *Able to Work*, Spinal Injuries Association, London.

Goffmann, E. (1963). *Stigma*, Prentice-Hall, Englewood Cliffs, New Jersey.

Gunn, S. L. and Peterson, C. A. (1978). Therapeutic recreation program design. Prentice-Hall, Englewood Cliffs, New Jersey.

Guttmann, L. (1976). *Textbook of Sport for the Disabled*, HM and M, Aylesbury.

Lawson, N. (1977). Significant events in a rehabilitation center: A multi-level longitudinal approach. Paper presented at the *American Congress of Rehabilitation Medicine, Miami Beach*. (Quoted in Trieschmann, 1980.)

Shearer, A. (1981). *Disability: Whose Handicap?* Blackwell, Oxford.

Taylor, G. (1967). Predicted versus actual response to spinal cord injury: a psychological study. Doctoral dissertation, University of Minnesota. (Quoted in Trieschmann, 1980.)

Trieschmann, R. B. (1980). *Spinal Cord Injuries — Psychological, Social and Vocational Adjustment*, Pergamon Press, Oxford and New York.

Postscript: The future

Rudy Capildeo and Audrey Maxwell

The theme of this book (and the series) is the approach of the rehabilitation team to a specific medical problem, in this instance, paraplegia. Almost every article published in recent years on current practice in medicine pays homage to the concept of 'team-work'. In practice, team-work remains the exception rather than the rule. Communication means meeting and talking to colleagues regularly, not on an ad hoc basis. The weekly meeting formalises communication between disciplines and is as important for the patient's sake as it is for members of the team. 'Too busy to attend a weekly meeting' is a nonsense, provided, of course, that there is only one major meeting a week for the team!

Since the pioneer work of Sir Ludwig Guttmann, a lot of progress has been made and due tribute to him and the members of his team at the National Spinal Injuries Unit, Stoke Mandeville Hospital, has been made throughout the book. This was the new beginning for paraplegic patients. Much work has yet to be done. Only the study of Jess Kraus and his colleagues (see Chapter 1) has tried to study the incidence of traumatic spinal cord injury. Similar prospective studies have yet to be done in the UK. The controversy of 'surgery versus no surgery' has yet to be resolved. The cause of heterotopic ossification is unknown and the treatment remains problematical. As in spasticity, prevention and medical treatment offer the best hope. Yet how much of the future in this subject depends upon improved road safety? The compulsory wearing of seat belts in cars is a beginning but it is not difficult to see how much work has yet to be done. The difficulty is how to do it.

The future as discussed by members of the rehabilitation team in this book (for example, Chapters 1 and 4) means the development of expertise on a local basis, in the district general hospital. The potential members of such a team are already there. It remains for the first meeting to be arranged. The assessment and subsequent rehabilitation of the spinal injuries victim in his own hospital and in his own community is a practical proposition and makes sound economic sense.

At the beginning of this book we mentioned the dreadful consequences of war and the inevitable casualties, particularly those with spinal injury. The possibility of war seems omnipresent. Developing further expertise in the rehabilitation of paraplegia will mean that the rehabilitation teams will be available if they are ever required.

Appendix 1: Useful addresses

HOUSING

Habinteg Housing Association,
6 Duke's Mews, Duke Street,
London W1
Tel.: 01-935 6931

Harewood Housing Society Ltd,
84 Bradford Road,
Otley, West Yorkshire LS21 3LE
Tel.: 09434 51879

Housing Corporation (Programme Division),
Maple House,
149 Tottenham Court Road,
London W1P 0BN
Tel.: 01-387 9466

John Grooms Housing Association,
10 Gloucester Drive,
Finsbury Park, London N4
Tel.: 01-802 7272

National Federation of Housing Associations,
30-32 Southampton Street,
London WC2E 7HE
Tel.: 01-240 2771

Raglan Housing Association,
Joliffe House,
West Street,
Poole, Dorset PH15 1LA
Tel.: 02013 78731

Shaftesbury Society Housing Association,
112 Regency Street,
London SW1
Tel.: 01-834 7581

HOUSING ORGANISATIONS – PRIVATE SECTOR

House Builders Federation,
82 New Cavendish Street,
London W1M 8AD
Tel.: 01-580 5588

National House-Building Council,
58 Portland Place,
London W1N 4BU
Tel.: 01-637 1248

GOVERNMENT DEPARTMENTS

Department of the Environment,
2 Marsham Street,
London SW1P 3EB
Tel.: 01-212 3434

DHSS,
Alexander Fleming House,
Elephant and Castle, London SE1 ODY
Tel.: 01-407 5522

Welsh Office,
Crown Buildings,
Cathays Park,
Cardiff, West Glamorgan CF1 3NA
Tel.: 0222 825111

Scottish Home and Health Department,
New St Andrew's House,
St James Centre,
Edinburgh EH1 3TF
Tel.: 031-556 8400

Department of Health and Social Services,
Dundonald House,
Upper Newtownards Road,
Belfast BT4 3SF
Tel.: 0232 650111

MOBILITY

Disabled Drivers' Association,
Ashwellthorpe,
Norwich, Norfolk NR16 1lEX
Tel.: 0508 41449

Disabled Drivers' Motor Club,
19 Dudley Gardens,
Ealing,
London W13 9LV
Tel.: 01-840 1515

Mobility Allowance Unit,
Warbreck Hill Road,
Blackpool FY2 OUZ
Tel.: 0253 52311

Mobility Information Service,
Copthorne Community Hall,
Shelton Road,
Shrewsbury, Shropshire SY3 8TD
Tel.: 0743 68383

Motobility,
Boundary House,
91–93 Charterhouse Street,
London EC1M 6BT
Tel.: 01-253 1211

Wheelchair Action,
2 Merthyr Terrace,
Barnes, London SW13 9DL
Tel.: 01-748 5574

TRAVEL

British Rail and Disabled Travellers,
British Railways Board (Central Publicity Unit),
Mulberry House,
Marylebone, London NW1
(British Rail publish a rail travel guide for the disabled,
which is available at local railway stations)

HOME AND HEALTH

The Association of Carers,
58 New Road,
Chatham, Kent ME4 4QR
Tel.: 0634 813981/2

Association of Crossroads Care Attendant Schemes Ltd,
Chief Executive Officer — Mrs Pat Osborne SRN, NCDN,
11 Whitehall Road,
Rugby, Warwickshire CV21 3AQ
Tel.: 0788 61536

Community Service Volunteers,
237 Pentonville Road,
London N1 9NJ
Tel.: 01-278 6601

Disabled Living Foundation,
346 Kensington High Street,
London W14 8NS
Tel.: 01-602 2491

Electronic Aids Loan Service for Disabled People,
Roger M. Jefcoate,
Willowbrook,
Swanbourne Road,
Mursley,
Milton Keynes, Bucks. MK17
Tel.: 0296 72533

Environment for the Handicapped,
126 Albert Street,
London NW1 7NE
Tel.: 01-482 2247

Holiday Care Service,
2 Old Bank Chambers,
Station Road,
Horley, Surrey RH6 9HW
Tel.: 02934 74535

Possum Users' Association,
14 Greenvale Drive,
Timsbury,
Nr. Bath, Avon BA3 1HP
Tel.: 0761 71184

Sexual Problems of the Disabled (SPOD),
The Diorama,
14 Peto Place,
London NW1 4DT
Tel.: 01-486 9823

WORK

Association of Disabled Professionals,
The Stables,
73 Pound Road,
Banstead, Surrey SM7 2HV
Tel.: 07373 52366

The British Computer Society,
13 Mansfield Street,
London W1M 0BP
Tel.: 01-637 0471

National Bureau for Handicapped Students,
40 Brunswick Square,
London WC1N 1AU
Tel.: 01-278 3459/3450

LEISURE

British Paraplegic Sports Society,
Ludwig Guttmann Sports Centre for the Disabled,
Harvey Road,
Stoke Mandeville,
Aylesbury, Bucks. HP21 8PP
Tel.: 0296 84848

British Sports Association for the Disabled,
Stoke Mandeville Stadium,
Harvey Road,
Aylesbury, Bucks. HP21 8PP
Tel.: 0296 27889

Gardens for the Disabled Trust,
Headcorn Manor,
Headcorn, Kent
Tel.: 0622 890360

Mouth and Foot Painting Artists,
9 Inverness Place,
London W2 3JF
Tel.: 01-229 4491

Open University,
Richard Tomlinson,
Disabled Students' Officer,
PO Box 48
Milton Keynes, Bucks. MK7 6AB

Photography for the Disabled,
190 Secrett House,
Ham Close,
Ham, Richmond, Surrey TW10 7PE
Tel.: 01-948 2342

Riding for the Disabled Association,
Avenue 'R',
National Agricultural Centre,

Kenilworth, Warwickshire CV8 2LY
Tel.: 0203 56107

WELFARE RIGHTS

Disability Alliance,
21 Star Street,
London W2 1QB
Tel.: 01-402 7026

Disablement Income Group (DIG),
Attlee House,
28 Commercial Street,
London E1 6LP
Tel.: 01-247 2128

VOLUNTARY ORGANISATIONS

Age Concern (England),
Bernard Sunley House,
60 Pitcairn Road,
Mitcham, Surrey, CR4 3LL
Tel.: 01-640 5431

Association of Crossroads Care Attendant Schemes Ltd,
11 Whitehall Road,
Rugby, Warwickshire CV21 3AQ
Tel.: 0788 61536

Community Service Volunteers,
237 Pentonville Road,
London N1 9NJ
Tel.: 01-278 6601

Dial UK,
Victoria Buildings,
117 High Street,
Clay Cross, Derbyshire
Tel.: 0246 864498

Leonard Cheshire Foundation,
26/29 Maunsel Street,
London SW1P 2QN
Tel.: 01-828 1822

Physically Handicapped & Able Bodied (PHAB),
42 Devonshire Street,
London W1N 1LN
Tel.: 01-637 7475

Royal Association for Disability and Rehabilitation (RADAR),
25 Mortimer Street,
London W1N 8AB
Tel.: 01-637 5400

Spinal Injuries Association,
5 Crowndale Road,
London NW1 1TU
Tel.: 01-388 6840

The Sue Ryder Foundation,
Cavendish,
Sudbury, Suffolk CO10 8AY
Tel.: 0787 280252/280653

Appendix 2: Useful publications

Designing for the Disabled, by S. Goldsmith,
Royal Institute of British Architects,
66 Portland Place,
London W1

*Directory for the Disabled: A Handbook of Information
and Opportunities for Disabled People*, by Ann
Darnborough and Derek Kinade (Woodhead-Faulkner,
Cambridge)

Disability Rights Handbook,
21 Star Street,
London W2 1QB
Tel.: 01-402 7026

Help for Handicapped People, Leaflet HB1, Department of
Health and Social Security

Motoring and Mobility,
RADAR,
25 Mortimer Street,
London W1N 8AB
Tel.: 01-637 5400

So You're Paralysed. . . , by Bernadette Fallon, and *Able to
Work*, by Bernadette Fallon,
Spinal Injuries Association,
5 Crowndale Road,
London NW1 1TU
Tel.. 01-388 6840

Author index

Subject index

Parasympathetic fibres 32
Pelvic floor 32
Pelvic nerve, stimulation of 43
Perineal muscles 31, 32
Perineal urethrostomy 40
Periurethral striated muscles,
    stimulation of 43
Phenoxybenzamine 39
Phentolamine 39
Phenylephrine 38
Physiotherapist 49, 51, 78, 116
Physiotherapy 5, 11, 52, 54
    aims of treatment 51
    in secondary prevention 56–58
Plastazote jacket 17
Plaster of Paris cast 14
Plastic surgery 24
Pneumatic Support Garment 53
Pneumothorax 7
Poliomyelitis 5
Posture 61
Pressure sores 8, 9, 13, 14, 17,
    18, 20, 56
    prevention of 22–23
    surgical repair of 24
    treatment of 23–24
Prognosis 10–12
    long-term 1
Propanolol 39
Prophylactic anticoagulation 8
Pudendal neurectomy 40
Pulmonary disease 10
Pulmonary embolism 8
Pyrazinamide 29
Pyridostigmine bromide 38

Quadriparesis 2, 4, 5
    prognosis 11
Quadriplegia 1, 2, 4, 5, 11, 78
    complete 11
    immediate outcome 10
    incomplete 11, *see also* Quadri-
        paresis
    prognosis 11
    see also Tetraplegia

Radiographic procedures 8

Radioisotope scanning 22
Radiologists 11
Radiology 35
Radiotherapy 7
α and β Receptors 38, 39
Record linkage 3
Recreation 128–131
Re-employment 62, 74
Rehabilitation 1, 3, 5, 10, 11,
    20, 51, 54, 55, 77
    aspects of 122–124
    employment 108–109
    physical 49, 50, 83–84
    social 61
    sport in 53
Rehabilitation team 18, 49,
    59–60, 61, 64, 78, 79, 83,
    89, 113, 133
    communication in 80, 133
    information from 81, 86
Rehabilitation units 3
Remploy 113
Renal failure 31, 47
    assessment 34–35
    diagnosis 34–35
Reticular formation 33
Renal function 35
Research 55
Reserpine 38
Resuscitation
    emergency 7
    initial 14
Ribs, fractured 7, 9
Rifampicin 29
Road traffic accidents 25
    see also Motor vehicle collisions
Robert Jones and Agnes Hunt
    Orthopaedic Hospital,
    Oswestry 58, 71
Royal Association for Disability
    and Rehabilitation 89

Sacral autonomic centre 32
Sacral block 40
Sacral ventral roots, stimulation
    of 43
Scoliosis 57